A ROW
A DAY
FOR
A YEAR

A ROW A DAY

FOR

A YEAR

Set a Goal—Track Your Progress

D.P. ORDWAY

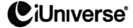

A ROW A DAY FOR A YEAR

iUniverse books may be ordered through booksellers or by contacting:

iUniverse
1663 Liberty Drive
Bloomington, IN 47403
www.iuniverse.com
1-800-Authors (1-800-288-4677)

ISBN: 978-1-4917-6135-9 (sc)
ISBN: 978-1-4917-6136-6 (e)

Library of Congress Control Number: 2015902782

Print information available on the last page.

iUniverse rev. date: 03/17/2015

"'Row Daily' should be handed to every person who wants to fall in love with indoor rowing. It is passion and knowledge at its best. This book ['A Row a Day'] is another great book and a great tool for indoor rowing people."

Santiago Fuentes. Dental Surgeon; National Champion Rower; Coaching, Regatta Management and other international experience for over 20 years, including referee, 2012 London Olympics and numerous other international regattas.

"We are relearning that moderate exercise keeps us healthy and helps us age well. Following the success of his first book on rowing as daily exercise, Dusty lays out a journal approach to capture daily entries, combined with advice on training programs, cross-training and stretching. The quotes scattered through the book from Plato and Seneca to President John Kennedy and the Merck manual are entertaining, inspiring, and full of common sense. A wonderful recipe for living better and rowing daily."

Joan W. Miller, MD. Chief of Ophthalmology, Mass Eye and Ear and Mass General Hospital. Chair, Department of Ophthalmology, Harvard Medical School. MIT Varsity Women's Crew, Captain, Boat Club Commodore and Straight T Award winner.

"Before I picked up 'Row Daily, Breathe Deeper, Live Better,' I was an intermittent exerciser. I was stuck. Despite my efforts, workouts had hit a plateau. Reading the book helped me realign my exercise goals. Now I work out 6 days a week. I feel better, my work on the erg has improved, and my cycling has improved, as well."

Dan Gallmeyer. Controls Engineer, 50s, no athletic background.

"When I first read 'Row Daily,' I had no interest in rowing or exercising every day. . . . I had always considered exercise as something to recover from, that it was necessary to take days of rest in between exercising. Last fall, as I considered how to get through another Michigan winter, I finally decided to get my own Concept2 rower. I have used it almost every day. My rowing sessions are like meditating with exercise. I listen to book recordings while I row, and some days I feel like I could keep going for hours. It has helped me to lose some pounds, helped to improve my posture and I feel much stronger."

Kris Estill. Automotive Engineering Process Analyst, 50s, occasional runner

"Dustin introduced me to indoor rowing (and sculling) years ago, when our sons were high school rowers and running was my main form of exercise. I purchased a Concept2 Model C rower primarily for my son's use. I used it at first for cross-training, finding that the handy little computer (then a PM-2) made it a convenient tool for high-intensity interval workouts. Also, I found the rowing machine useful for maintaining my conditioning while I was in rehab for my seemingly endless series of running-related injuries.
"I finally got tired of all the injuries and took up biking. But, since I live in Michigan and don't enjoy cold weather biking, indoor rowing has become the mainstay of my year-round exercise program. It

is convenient and an efficient way to maintain my fitness for some of the longer bike rides I like to do. The combination of biking and rowing has left me essentially free of exercise-related injuries."
Todd Dickinson. Attorney, 50s, former runner and cyclist

"'Row Daily' has been an essential part of our indoor rowing curriculum. Students don't just learn the basics of indoor rowing technique - they really start to internalize the many health (and other) benefits of rowing, indoors and out. Sure, it helps that the text is clearly written and easy to understand. But the real power of this book is Dustin's ability to engage students from the pages, leading them through a variety of experiences and building healthy habits that extend well outside of the erg room."
Landon Bartley. President, Grand Rapids Rowing Association

"I first took up rowing as an undergraduate at MIT in the late '60s. Our coach gave the new recruits an old magazine article, 'The Eight-Oared Shell', written by Oliver La Farge, that movingly reflected the feeling that I later experienced in competitive rowing: 'You have known complete exertion, you have answered every trouble of mind, spirit and being with skilled violence and guided unrestraint, a complete happiness with eight other men over a short stretch of water has brought you catharsis.' *I continued to row competitively and internationally into the 90's. I no longer row regularly but still can't pass a body of water without reminiscing on the pleasure of my past early morning rows on the peaceful waters of the Charles River in Boston and the River Thames in England. And, I still look back, with as much satisfaction as any other experience in my life, on the times when I and the men in our boat achieved that catharsis in victory. I still enjoy regular exercise and can credit that, among other things, with being still within a few pounds of being a lightweight."*
John M. Malarkey, Managing Director with Bechtel Enterprises; member of MIT lightweight eight that competed at the Henley Royal Regatta in 1969 and U.S. lightweight eight that competed in the European Championships in Moscow in 1973.

"Books like 'Row Daily' get me off my chair and into action. Stress is common in my life. Exercise makes it manageable. Exercise is my silver bullet! Life is so much more enjoyable. I never think 'Oh I've got to do this . . .,' but how can I do more. There is so much joy, I feel like a kid again. I plan to exercise daily for the rest of my life."
Jack Acheff. late 50s, computer programmer whose goal is a 100k row.

To the rowers in my family
And to the family of rowers.

Acknowledgements

Thanks to the many people who have responded positively and with suggestions and criticisms to "Row Daily, Breathe Deeper, Live Better: A Guide to Moderate Exercise." To my surprise and pleasure, members of the rowing community, the coaches and competitors who experience rowing as a highly competitive sport, have not challenged the concept that anyone can enjoy rowing as a form of daily moderate exercise, even though it does not fulfil the fundamental rowing precept of pushing one's limits. Nor have they pushed back with the argument that moderate rowing is not real rowing. That open-minded response may well be the second stage of the rowing revolution that began nearly 50 years ago with the development of quality indoor rowing machines everyone can use.

Cover photo courtesy of WaterRower. Author photo by Gary Howe.

"If I'd known I was gonna live this long,
I'd have taken better care of myself."
Eubie Blake at age 100

"Moderate exercise, preferably every day,
provides significant health benefits."
Merck Manual of Health and Aging, at 806

"Eighty percent of success is showing up."
Woody Allen

"All parts of the body which have a function,
if used in moderation and exercised in labors in which each is accustomed,
become thereby healthy, well developed and age more slowly,
but if unused they become liable to disease, defective in growth and age quickly."
Hippocrates

"One run, on one weekend, justifies existence."
103-year old skier Lou Batori (2014)

"Your body takes care of itself for the first fifty years.
After that, you have to make an effort."
Nick Hanson to Mike Daley over wine and scampi
at San Francisco's Caffe Sport,
S. Siegel, Judgment Day (MacAdam/Cage 2008), at 173.

Contents

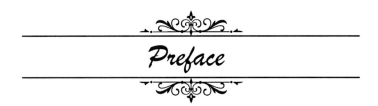

Preface

This book is my challenge to you to row every day for a year and see how great you feel.

We have a growing population of what used to be called the elderly. In my view, the former meaning of the word "elderly" must be discarded. Those who choose to remain sedentary may stick with the old definition if they wish. The rest of us should change it; we have learned that exercise helps improve health, prolong life and reduce the effects of aging. We can remain more fit and active well into the years that used to be a time of slow decay unto death. Politicians can fight over health insurance. Medical researchers can continue to develop cures for cancer and other diseases and physical ills, as we all are at risk. In the meantime, we 'non-elderly' can enjoy the benefits of the body's miraculous, adaptive regenerative power through exercise.

Few people row every day. Highly trained athletes plan rest into their calendars. They do that because they are so fit and work so hard that they sometimes exercise to exhaustion. Their extreme effort may involve depleting their muscles' stores of energy, for example. Exhaustion may also stem from strength-building exercises done at an intensity that requires time for muscle recovery. The need for a rest day may arise when a very fit person pushes the anaerobic threshold to a point far beyond the "ordinary" person's capacity to "drain" the body. That extreme level of exercise (and corresponding rest) can be a great tool for the competitive athlete working toward peak performance. The highly trained athlete who has pushed her limits to that degree needs rest to allow the body to recover in order to grow stronger. It is the same principle of demand and response, the body's adaptation to stimulus, but taken to a different level than an ordinarily-fit person normally will experience or achieve.

Since I am not a believer that people are divided in "ordinary" and "extraordinary" sub-classes, let me explain the preceding reference to the limited capacity of an ordinary person to drain the body of strength and energy. Put simply, whatever your genetic makeup, you have to be exceptionally fit to push yourself to your limits. Someone who is not so exceptionally fit will tire before she can drain her reserves of energy and require additional time and rest for her body to recover. That feeling of being tired is not the same as the fatigue of an exceptionally fit athlete. Anyone can become extraordinarily fit. However, the simple truth is that most of us most of the time are not that fit. And if you are not that well-conditioned, you will find that you will stop exercising long before you reach the point of exhaustion or depletion that requires adding rest of more than 24 hours to your exercise regimen. You may feel tired when you complete your daily row. But you are not likely to be in that deep a 'trough,' that completely drained. You will recover more quickly than the super-fit athlete for the simple reason that your feeling of exhaustion is based on a limited perception of what is normal energy use and manageable bodily fatigue.

Obviously, although I am attributing the sense of fatigue in most of us most of the time to a subjective sense that is disassociated from our true limits when we are exceptionally fit, fatigue is not just subjective. First, the feeling of being tired is real and it is important to acknowledge that feeling. I do not suggest overdoing your moderate exercise on the theory that your sense of fatigue is kicking in artificially early. Do not ignore what you feel. It is real for you. Second, the sense of fatigue may represent some aspect of your present bodily condition that reflects a training state or recovery condition akin to the highly trained athlete's drained system. Thus, if for some reason (*e.g.,* illness, muscle soreness) you feel depleted and you find your body is not recovering by the time of your next daily row, take a longer rest and/or a restful recovery row.

The average person, novice rower and non-rower alike, is more likely to try for three or four workouts per week rather than seven. Why promote daily exercise? The reason is simply that when one exercises moderately, the more the better. The body functions on a daily cycle; use it. But also consider this viewpoint: The body functions better at a higher level than when it is at rest. From another angle, one might say, being physically at rest really is for rest and is not the preferred normal level of physical activity for a healthy body; it is preferable to move. Having said that, even if your pace or energy output is moderate, if you continue long enough you may begin to leave the range of moderation and achieve an extreme outcome.

One new rower contacted me about his desire to row three hours at a time. He had done other endurance sports, was working hard, and had some aches and pains he wondered about. Eventually, he got past that phase and worked up to rowing a marathon distance (over 42 kilometers) at one time. But that came after he took into account the need to balance different types of workouts and to rest when he felt so depleted in muscle strength that he was weak the following day. In short, that level of fatigue is possible in an 'ordinary' person, even though it is rare. The benefits of daily exercise are especially clear for the average person of years. Many of the quotations included here are from the medical profession. They remind us in many ways that the greatest health benefits come from the moderate exercise we all can do, and that the benefits are many, regardless of age and other conditions.

Take the challenge; try to row every day for a year. Whether or not you succeed in rowing every day, you likely will exercise more consistently than you have before. That will be good for your fitness. Equally important, it can be good for your health. The ability of the human body to function more effectively through exercise and thereby naturally to enhance our health can help us live longer and with more enjoyment.

Some may wonder, is this magic? Certainly, I would say, *there is magic here* in the sense that the human body has incredible self-healing and self-improvement powers. When you exercise, your body responds by strengthening itself for the next day. Somehow, that natural and automatic response either causes or goes hand in hand with other benefits such as helping the body to avoid or fight disease.

On the other hand, we should be clear that *there no magic here* in two important senses:

- First, there is no incantation or spell with an automatic or guaranteed outcome. That is, while I am convinced that daily exercise can help us all fight most forms of ill health, from the common cold to cancer, each of us has our own history, our own genetic makeup, our own habits, our own chemical environment, our own starting point, our own risks. Exercise is no guarantee, but consider it an ally.
- Second, you have to get yourself onto that rowing machine each day to get the benefits. Exercise does not guarantee you will live to the age of 100 and be healthy and moving yourself about at that time, but it does improve your chances if you make the effort each day to harness the body's capability to adapt.

Try it! See how your year goes. Enjoy what it does for you today and, I hope, for years to come.

D.P. Ordway

Introduction

There is little that motivates people more than setting a goal and monitoring progress. This rowing journal is set up to make it easier for you to keep track of your progress and to encourage you to set goals for yourself.

The first goal is the simplest–row daily. Once you have decided to try to row daily, you will succeed more than before at exercising each day. That, in turn, as we are told by the medical profession, will have a positive effect on your health as well as your fitness. But rowing for a year and improving health are long term goals that will tend to accrue in small steps; you may not notice specific changes day to day or even week to week. On the other hand, you will also find that you can help achieve the goal of rowing each day by setting short term goals that include specific expectations, whether for speed, time, distance or a new activity.

As you begin to think more long term by focusing on what your progress will be for a year, consider an even longer definition of long term. Consider the duration of your life. Twenty year olds think they will live forever; at least, they act if they do and normally would not think about the duration. Thirty and forty year olds are often too busy to think about more than the present, or so it often seems. But once we reach our fifties and sixties, our thoughts at some point will turn naturally to whether we are past the middle of the game. It may be tempting to anticipate the end. Consider instead anticipating continuing to play the game and enjoying yourself until the end.

This book is not intended to replace directions you receive from a coach, rowing instructor or experienced friend about establishing an exercise routine for yourself. Nor is it intended to provide all the pieces you would want or need to develop a routine on your own. The limited information about training ideas and regimens is included at the back of the book purposely; that information is supplemental to the two central points that (1) just rowing each day is in itself an achievement and (2) your best guide to developing a plan for yourself may be your own experience.

Do what works for you.

Do what fits your schedule and background.

Do what your attention to your daily rowing tells you will work for your body.

Do what you enjoy.

Some notes on how this book is set up:

- First, because you may start using the entry spaces of the log at any time of year, each month has 31 days worth of entries.
- Second, each month has extra spaces for additional workouts. Anyone may exercise more than 31 times per month because it is often useful to exercise more than once in a day.
- Third, do not limit yourself to reading through "A Row a Day" in order as the year goes by. Each month begins with a short note that may be useful to you at any time of year in connection with your personal exercise routine. Browsing through the book may help you plan your exercise more usefully than reading it a month at a time as the year goes by.
- Fourth, at the end of each month is a short summary page where you can keep track of your progress. In an ideal world, that page would be where you would record your perfect attendance of daily exercise. In the real world, it is a place to recap your level of success at trying to exercise daily. Look at your results from different perspectives; see which you find most satisfying and encouraging.
- At the end of each season is a different summary page that may assist you in looking back in order to inform how you plan ahead. Did you set goals? What were they? What happened with your efforts to achieve your goals? What will your new goal(s) be?
- Quotations from a variety of sources are included at the start of each month for two reasons, entertainment and education. Most of us do not fully appreciate the extent to which we harm ourselves through a sedentary lifestyle, or how much we can help ourselves through daily, moderate exercise. The point is not to be athletic or to be like someone else. The point is to use your body's natural sustaining and self-healing powers. The medical profession is way ahead of most of us in acknowledging the extraordinary positive health effects of moderate exercise. They may not understand fully how it works, but they know it does work. If there is key substantive content in this book, you might say it is in these quotations. Consider the quotes the bull's-eye of the imaginary target that guides your development of a daily routine. Your goals, how you track your progress and your daily efforts may represent the outer rings of the target that build on the bull's-eye.
- At the back of the book are several appendices with information you may find useful as you plan your rows. Just as "Row Daily" offered input on stretching and core work but did not set forth a detailed plan, the information in these appendices is input for you to consider rather than direction for you to follow. It is intended to be introductory input for someone who is not a trained athlete, someone who does not have a personal trainer or coach to guide her. It is not intended to be complete or to set forth a routine. I assume you may have begun rowing in an unstructured mode, rowing as if you were going for a walk, without goal or direction. The small amount of information in the appendices may help the beginner who wants to plan to decide what she would like to do the next day and the day after that. A regimen would require adherence. With this limited input, you are free to exercise your choice according to your personal preferences

for your daily rows. For those who would prefer a directive to row a specific workout each day, forgive my pushing back and placing the control in your hands.

You may hesitate to set a goal or keep track of your progress for fear of failure. To some, calculating and recording a less than perfect score may seem discouraging. To me, it is just the opposite. Engaging in any exercise today is a plus compared to doing none. How many pluses can you accumulate? By looking back at the end of each month at the ratio of days you exercise to those you skip or miss, you will see success with every active day. You will develop a pattern of that success you can compare as the months go by.

It may help you to imagine three people - Ron, Melanie (Mel) and Andrea (Andie) as fellow rowers. You can compare their situations to yours. What differences do their lifestyle choices make in how their bodies function, and does that inform your choices?

- *Ron is in his late 50s and has rowed and competed for years. To his friends, it seems rowing is Ron's first interest, the activity by which everything else in his life is regulated. He works out virtually every day. He has a year-round plan for training. He lives on a lake where he can row every morning and has his own indoor rowing machine. He belongs to a local health club where he can lift weights and use other aerobic equipment. He competes (and medals) year after year at many regattas. He enjoys coaching. He is constantly trying to learn ways to be more effective, including managing his diet to support his desire to be fit and fast.*
- *Mel is in her mid-40s and leads a sedentary life. She commutes by car. If she needs milk or eggs, she drives to the store. Her home is not close to her office, the pharmacy, or other places she goes every day. At work, she sits at a desk with a computer. At home, she has hobbies that involving sitting and working with her hands. She likes to read and watches some television. Mel is not totally inactive physically. She lives in a two-story house, so she walks up and down the stairs every day. She enjoys gardening. She occasionally takes a walk. She enjoys sunning and swimming at the beach in the summer. But she has not previously engaged in regular planned exercise, attended aerobics classes, jogged regularly, gone for bike rides, or planned any other exercise activity on a daily basis.*
- *Andie is a year older than Mel and exercises regularly. Andie's life is similar to Mel's, including commuting by train, working at a desk, and living in an apartment (she takes an elevator to her fifth floor apartment). However, Andie tries to exercise regularly, and succeeds on average five to six days a week. Her favorite activities are cycling, spinning, rowing and cross-country skiing. But she also periodically will take 'muscle pump' weight lifting classes at the gym and yoga classes at a local strip mall yoga center. Andie also sometimes plans vacations organized around exercise, such as attending rowing regattas or hiking or bicycling in Europe.*

Consider what differences there may be going on physiologically inside Ron, Mel and Andie's bodies, in how their lungs, hearts, organs, bones, joints, skin, and digestive systems function. Assume all three are healthy, with no condition that is an obvious precursor to disease and no disease presently known to be threatening or afflicting them. Consider how the differences in their lifestyles might affect the parts of their bodies and how those parts will perform for them over the next 10-30 years.

This log does not attempt to answer these questions. But one purpose is to encourage you to ask yourself what is happening inside your body as you exercise (or not) each day. How does your body feel? How do you feel? Does your exercise affect how you feel during the rest of the day and night?

Another purpose of this log is to make it easier to exercise regularly by providing a log format that focuses on two things that may be different from the records a training competitor keeps. Record here (1) whether or not you exercised and (2) your observations about how you felt. Your primary focus with this log is not output (speed, time or distance rowed) but participation. If you wish, you can include data, as well.

The end of each season in the log provides space for a recap on scoring, goal-setting, and injecting variety into your exercise routine. I have purposely limited the content that provides direction as your attention, your choices and what you learn from them are more important. What you observe as you row, what you notice because you are keeping track, and – most importantly – the effects on your body, are the things this book is really all about.

D.P. Ordway
dpordway@rowdaily.com
www.rowdaily.com

January

"Those who think they have not time for bodily exercise will sooner or later have to find time for illness."

Edward Stanley, Earl of Derby (1826-93) (12/20/1873 address at Liverpool College)

"Take care of your body with steadfast fidelity. The soul must see through these eyes alone, and if they are dim, the whole world is clouded."

Goethe

"Exercise – physical activity done regularly—is something people can and should do for a lifetime. It helps people feel and function better physically and mentally. It also helps reduce the risk of many disorders."

Mark H. Beers, MD, Ed in Chief, *The Merck Manual of Health and Aging* (2004) ("Merck"), at 805.

"A lack of activity destroys the good condition of every human being while movement and methodical physical exercise save and preserve it."

Plato

"If you look at the lowest quintile of fitness, those are the people who account for the bulk of the mortality risk. The mortality difference between average fitness and good and excellent fitness is really very small."

Michael Lauer, MD (Cleveland Clinic cardiologist), in Kolata, Gina. *Ultimate Fitness: The Quest for Truth about Exercise and Health.* (2003) ("Kolata"), at 64.

"There is a simple, basic fact about exercise and your health: fitness cuts your risk of dying. . . . Couch potatoes are now being grouped with cigarette smokers as taking their lives into their own hands. . . . The more frequent the exercise, the greater the benefit, but you don't have to overdo it. Moderate exercise . . . proved to be nearly as protective as vigorous exercise."

John W. Rowe, MD, and Robert L. Kahn, Ph.D., *Successful Aging* (1998) ("Successful Aging"), at 6.

January – Take an Indoor Rowing Class

If you are a beginning rower, you have a lot to gain from taking a rowing class. You will learn about the machine, how to row efficiently, and more ways to use the machine effectively for your own health and fitness. Even if you are an experienced rower, you may learn a great deal that helps you row for health by taking a class. Those who have taught themselves to row will be able to correct mistakes. Those who have competitive rowing experience may learn that using the erg does not have to mean experiencing pain. If you took a learn-to-row class on the water, you may find that an indoor rowing class can help answer your questions about the stroke and teach you new ways to improve your technique.

There are many opportunities to participate in an indoor rowing class. Some rowing clubs and associations offer indoor rowing classes in the winter, when they cannot offer learn to row classes on the river. They may offer them at other times of year, too. Some personal trainers offer individual sessions and group classes year round. Health facilities focused on rowing hold regular sessions. And general fitness clubs may offer occasional rowing classes. If you use a gym that has a couple ergs but does not offer classes, ask about it.

Many indoor rowing classes are guided workouts. You show up at the appointed time and enjoy a workout session simply by following the trainer in the front of the room. But for those seeking to learn more about rowing, most facilities and trainers who offer workouts will also provide rowing lessons.

What, you may ask, can you learn in a rowing class? Here are some of the types of lessons you can hope to learn through indoor rowing classes.

Introductory classes: In a class designed for beginners, you can expect to review the basics of the rowing motion, including the terminology. These basic skills will help you use rowing for health and fitness on your own. And they will make it easier to learn more. You will learn about the rowing machine, including how to care for it and how to use it safely and efficiently. Although key components of rowing on the water in a shell (such as timing, balance and interaction with moving water) are missing on the rowing machine, there is a great deal you can learn on the erg that will help you later if you try rowing outdoors. Your introductory class may be set up and conducted with that in mind so that what you learn indoors in January helps you when you first get in a boat in the spring or summer.

Intermediate classes can help you improve your rowing in a number of ways. Whereas the introductory classes probably did not show you ways to row harder, an intermediate class may be designed to help you understand how the same rowing that offers you a tool for basic fitness can be used to improve your fitness. The process of working harder also creates a very useful dynamic for improving your technique. The reason is simple: As we work harder, errors become evident that may not show up when 'paddling' lightly or rowing easily. For example, as you row harder, small muscles will tend to tighten up and tire before the larger muscle groups. That leads to technique problems that become more evident in an intermediate context. Once they are more obvious, it is easier to work on them and correct them. And by correcting them you enhance your ability to get better exercise comfortably.

An intermediate class may also provide more guidance on using the erg monitor, clock, your pulse and other forms of input to guide and/or track your workout. While the beginner class may not result in your breathing much more deeply and becoming winded, an intermediate class ought to give you that opportunity to learn more about the boundaries of your comfort level using your breathing. You may even do some baseline pieces of different distances or times to set you up for personal record keeping. Learning to use additional training tools will enrich your experience.

Advanced erg classes will likely be focused on training for competition or for more enhanced fitness improvement. You will always return to the use of good technique. However, your time will be spent mostly on tools you can use to improve your performance during practice so that you can maximize your performance in a race or to meet a goal. Training regimens can vary with your personal choices, but understanding and trying different workouts can give you tools you can use on your own. This can be useful even if you do not intend to race; the same range of workout options can enhance your enjoyment of rowing for health, general fitness and longevity.

Ron no longer takes rowing classes. He has taught many himself to adults and juniors, both on the water and indoors. He is more likely to discuss rowing technique and training choices with fellow competitors in order to add to the continual improvement he applies to his year-round training regimen.

Mel has never rowed. She can act on her New Year's resolution by signing up for an introductory rowing class. This year, one of the local rowing associations is holding classes at the downtown YWCA.

Andie has taken learn-to-row classes in the past and has a late-winter ski vacation planned up north where the snow will be reliable, she hopes, for cross-country skiing. She checks the local listings and signs up for an intermediate rowing class just to see what she can learn and to take a break from the Yoga and Pilates classes she has attended during the last several months.

1

Date, day, time, location: _____

Feeling of energy/health before: _____ *during:* _____ *after:* _____

Challenges: _____

Max effort/breathing/pulse: _____

Core: _____

Stretching: _____

Successes: _____

Other: _____

Time/Distance/Totals, if any: _____

2

Date, day, time, location: _____

Feeling of energy/health before: _____ *during:* _____ *after:* _____

Challenges: _____

Max effort/breathing/pulse: _____

Core: _____

Stretching: _____

Successes: _____

Other: _____

Time/Distance/Totals, if any: _____

3

Date, day, time, location: _____

Feeling of energy/health before: _____ *during:* _____ *after:* _____

Challenges: _____

Max effort/breathing/pulse: _____

Core: _____

Stretching: _____

Successes: _____

Other: _____

Time/Distance/Totals, if any: _____

4

Date, day, time, location: _____

Feeling of energy/health before: _____ *during:* _____ *after:* _____

Challenges: _____

Max effort/breathing/pulse: _____

Core: _____

Stretching: _____
Successes: _____
Other: _____
Time/Distance/Totals, if any: _____

5

Date, day, time, location: _____
Feeling of energy/health before: _____*during:*_____ *after:* _____
Challenges: _____
Max effort/breathing/pulse: _____
Core: _____
Stretching: _____
Successes: _____
Other: _____
Time/Distance/Totals, if any: _____

6

Date, day, time, location: _____
Feeling of energy/health before: _____*during:*_____ *after:* _____
Challenges: _____
Max effort/breathing/pulse: _____
Core: _____
Stretching: _____
Successes: _____
Other: _____
Time/Distance/Totals, if any: _____

7

Date, day, time, location: _____
Feeling of energy/health before: _____*during:*_____ *after:* _____
Challenges: _____
Max effort/breathing/pulse: _____
Core: _____
Stretching: _____
Successes: _____
Other: _____
Time/Distance/Totals, if any: _____

What shall I do today . . . heute . . . hoy . . . aujourd'hui . . . oggi . . . idag . . . tanaan . . . avui . . .

8

Date, day, time, location: _____
Feeling of energy/health before: _____during:_____ after: _____
Challenges: _____
Max effort/breathing/pulse: _____
Core: _____
Stretching: _____
Successes: _____
Other: _____
Time/Distance/Totals, if any: _____

9

Date, day, time, location: _____
Feeling of energy/health before: _____during:_____ after: _____
Challenges: _____
Max effort/breathing/pulse: _____
Core: _____
Stretching: _____
Successes: _____
Other: _____
Time/Distance/Totals, if any: _____

10

Date, day, time, location: _____
Feeling of energy/health before: _____during:_____ after: _____
Challenges: _____
Max effort/breathing/pulse: _____
Core: _____
Stretching: _____
Successes: _____
Other: _____
Time/Distance/Totals, if any: _____

11

Date, day, time, location: _____
Feeling of energy/health before: _____during:_____ after: _____
Challenges: _____
Max effort/breathing/pulse: _____
Core: _____

Stretching: _____

Successes: _____

Other: _____

Time/Distance/Totals, if any: _____

12

Date, day, time, location: _____

Feeling of energy/health before: _____ *during:* _____ *after:* _____

Challenges: _____

Max effort/breathing/pulse: _____

Core: _____

Stretching: _____

Successes: _____

Other: _____

Time/Distance/Totals, if any: _____

13

Date, day, time, location: _____

Feeling of energy/health before: _____ *during:* _____ *after:* _____

Challenges: _____

Max effort/breathing/pulse: _____

Core: _____

Stretching: _____

Successes: _____

Other: _____

Time/Distance/Totals, if any: _____

14

Date, day, time, location: _____

Feeling of energy/health before: _____ *during:* _____ *after:* _____

Challenges: _____

Max effort/breathing/pulse: _____

Core: _____

Stretching: _____

Successes: _____

Other: _____

Time/Distance/Totals, if any: _____

What shall I do today . . . heute . . . hoy . . . aujourd'hui . . . oggi . . . idag . . . tanaan . . . avui . . .

15

Date, day, time, location: _____

Feeling of energy/health before: _____ *during:* _____ *after:* _____

Challenges: _____

Max effort/breathing/pulse: _____

Core: _____

Stretching: _____

Successes: _____

Other: _____

Time/Distance/Totals, if any: _____

16

Date, day, time, location: _____

Feeling of energy/health before: _____ *during:* _____ *after:* _____

Challenges: _____

Max effort/breathing/pulse: _____

Core: _____

Stretching: _____

Successes: _____

Other: _____

Time/Distance/Totals, if any: _____

17

Date, day, time, location: _____

Feeling of energy/health before: _____ *during:* _____ *after:* _____

Challenges: _____

Max effort/breathing/pulse: _____

Core: _____

Stretching: _____

Successes: _____

Other: _____

Time/Distance/Totals, if any: _____

18

Date, day, time, location: _____

Feeling of energy/health before: _____ *during:* _____ *after:* _____

Challenges: _____

Max effort/breathing/pulse: _____

Core: _____

Stretching: _____
Successes: _____
Other: _____
Time/Distance/Totals, if any: _____

19

Date, day, time, location: _____
Feeling of energy/health before: _____*during:*_____ *after:* _____
Challenges: _____
Max effort/breathing/pulse: _____
Core: _____
Stretching: _____
Successes: _____
Other: _____
Time/Distance/Totals, if any: _____

20

Date, day, time, location: _____
Feeling of energy/health before: _____*during:*_____ *after:* _____
Challenges: _____
Max effort/breathing/pulse: _____
Core: _____
Stretching: _____
Successes: _____
Other: _____
Time/Distance/Totals, if any: _____

21

Date, day, time, location: _____
Feeling of energy/health before: _____*during:*_____ *after:* _____
Challenges: _____
Max effort/breathing/pulse: _____
Core: _____
Stretching: _____
Successes: _____
Other: _____
Time/Distance/Totals, if any: _____

22

Date, day, time, location: _____

Feeling of energy/health before: _____*during:*_____ *after:* _____

Challenges: _____

Max effort/breathing/pulse: _____

Core: _____

Stretching: _____

Successes: _____

Other: _____

Time/Distance/Totals, if any: _____

23

Date, day, time, location: _____

Feeling of energy/health before: _____*during:*_____ *after:* _____

Challenges: _____

Max effort/breathing/pulse: _____

Core: _____

Stretching: _____

Successes: _____

Other: _____

Time/Distance/Totals, if any: _____

24

Date, day, time, location: _____

Feeling of energy/health before: _____*during:*_____ *after:* _____

Challenges: _____

Max effort/breathing/pulse: _____

Core: _____

Stretching: _____

Successes: _____

Other: _____

Time/Distance/Totals, if any: _____

25

Date, day, time, location: _____

Feeling of energy/health before: _____*during:*_____ *after:* _____

Challenges: _____

Max effort/breathing/pulse: _____

Core: _____

Stretching: _____

Successes: _____ . _____

Other: _____

Time/Distance/Totals, if any: _____

26

Date, day, time, location: _____

Feeling of energy/health before: _____*during:*_____ *after:* _____

Challenges: _____

Max effort/breathing/pulse: _____

Core: _____

Stretching: _____

Successes: _____

Other: _____

Time/Distance/Totals, if any: _____

27

Date, day, time, location: _____

Feeling of energy/health before: _____*during:*_____ *after:* _____

Challenges: _____

Max effort/breathing/pulse: _____

Core: _____

Stretching: _____

Successes: _____

Other: _____

Time/Distance/Totals, if any: _____

28

Date, day, time, location: _____

Feeling of energy/health before: _____*during:*_____ *after:* _____

Challenges: _____

Max effort/breathing/pulse: _____

Core: _____

Stretching: _____

Successes: _____

Other: _____

Time/Distance/Totals, if any: _____

29

Date, day, time, location: _____

Feeling of energy/health before: _____*during:*_____ *after:* _____

Challenges: _____

Max effort/breathing/pulse: _____

Core: _____

Stretching: _____

Successes: _____

Other: _____

Time/Distance/Totals, if any: _____

30

Date, day, time, location: _____

Feeling of energy/health before: _____*during:*_____ *after:* _____

Challenges: _____

Max effort/breathing/pulse: _____

Core: _____

Stretching: _____

Successes: _____

Other: _____

Time/Distance/Totals, if any: _____

31

Date, day, time, location: _____

Feeling of energy/health before: _____*during:*_____ *after:* _____

Challenges: _____

Max effort/breathing/pulse: _____

Core: _____

Stretching: _____

Successes: _____

Other: _____

Time/Distance/Totals, if any: _____

Extra Workouts 1

Date, day, time, location: _____

Feeling of energy/health before: _____during:_____ after: _____

Challenges: _____

Max effort/breathing/pulse: _____

Core: _____

Stretching: _____

Successes: _____

Other: _____

Time/Distance/Totals, if any: _____

Extra 2

Date, day, time, location: _____

Feeling of energy/health before: _____during:_____ after: _____

Challenges: _____

Max effort/breathing/pulse: _____

Core: _____

Stretching: _____

Successes: _____

Other: _____

Time/Distance/Totals, if any: _____

Extra 3

Date, day, time, location: _____

Feeling of energy/health before: _____during:_____ after: _____

Challenges: _____

Max effort/breathing/pulse: _____

Core: _____

Stretching: _____

Successes: _____

Other: _____

Time/Distance/Totals, if any: _____

Extra 4

Date, day, time, location: _____

Feeling of energy/health before: _____during:_____ after: _____

Challenges: _____

Max effort/breathing/pulse: _____

Core: _____

What shall I do today . . . heute . . . hoy . . . aujourd'hui . . . oggi . . . idag . . . tanaan . . . avui . . .

Stretching: _____

Successes: _____

Other: _____

Time/Distance/Totals, if any: _____

Extra 5

Date, day, time, location: _____

Feeling of energy/health before: _____*during:*_____ *after:* _____

Challenges: _____

Max effort/breathing/pulse: _____

Core: _____

Stretching: _____

Successes: _____

Other: _____

Time/Distance/Totals, if any: _____

End of Month Scoring

Method One: Basic (Number of days I exercised this month):_____
    Ultimate Goal: Every Day
    My Goal for This Month Was: _____
    My Goal for Next Month Is: _____
Method Two: Subtraction (Days I Rowed Minus Days Not):_____
    Initial Goal: Exceed Zero (row at least half the days)
    Ultimate Goal: Same as days in the month.
    My Goal for This Month Was: _____
    My Goal for Next Month Is: _____
Method Three: Division (Percentage = Days Rowed Divided by Total Days): _____
    Ultimate Goal: 100%
    My Goal for This Month Was:_____
    My Goal for Next Month Is: _____

Other Scores and Data for Month (Goals set and met; Times rowed; Distances rowed; Other):

_____

_____

_____

_____

_____

_____

_____

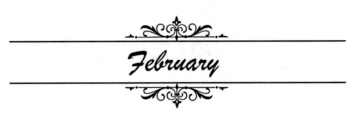

February

"*Today I broke my world record by three seconds. What I was trying to do was to break 8:00 [minutes for 2k], but I didn't quite manage it, but that leaves me something to look forward to. Although I don't know, at 81 years old I think that you're supposed to be going downhill instead of uphill, but we can keep trying.*"
   Joe Clinard, 2000 C.R.A.S.H.-B. Competitor

"*Intellectual tasting of life will not supersede muscular activity.*"
   Ralph Waldo Emerson

"*If you look at body fat, it seems to increase with age, even though your weight does not. That's a physiological fact of aging, they say. Heck it is. It is an adaptive effect of aging.*"

"*I have broadened the fitness concept to make it one of moderation and balance.*"

"*The reason I exercise is for the quality of life I enjoy.*"
   Dr. Kenneth H. Cooper

"*The improvement in cardiovascular fitness is clearly worth the effort, given that exercise slows the age-related decline in functional capacity and, quite possibly, increases active life expectancy.*"
   John Zumerchik, Editor, *Encyclopedia of Sports Science*, Volume 2, (1997) ("Encyclopedia"), at 593-9

"*[T]he benefits of exercise even go so far as to negate the adverse effects of other risk factors, such as smoking, high blood pressure, and high blood sugar! . . . This dominant effect of fitness over other risk factors . . . makes physical fitness perhaps the single most important thing an older person can do to remain healthy. Physical activity is at the crux of successful aging . . . . If you are at risk because of certain habits you cannot change, getting in good physical shape is one valuable step you can take to keep yourself alive longer.*"
   Successful Aging, at 137

February – Train to Race; Train to Improve

The tools a competitive rower uses to prepare to race are useful for the everyday rower, as well. They include double workouts (exercising two times per day), weight lifting, core exercises, and cross-training such as cycling. While the competitor may be using these tools to achieve optimum fitness or to prepare for maximum effort for a personal best performance, you can also use them at your own pace to enhance your rowing for health. For example, you can use double workouts to incorporate cross-training, continuing your daily rows while adding a different type of exercise at another time of day. A competitor may lift weights using a regimen of many different lifts and push to her limits; you can lift weights in a more focused and limited way to improve your strength in key muscle groups. And, if you are just beginning or out of shape, you can use weight lifting judiciously to begin to add tone and strength to muscles that you have become accustomed not to using.

When training to race, you will identify your goals well in advance; use the competition date to work backwards to plan your workouts; set a realistic target for your time in the race; and use that target in comparison to your current status to develop a plan to build up your fitness and speed over time. If you are using a race for the first time as a target to enhance your workouts, think in advance about your schedule and other activities (work, family obligations, vacations, other travel, and so on) and be realistic about the time you have to train. Plan to get more sleep and to eat better. Identify any related goals you have besides your race time, such as whether you intend to lose weight, increase the weight you can lift, achieve related goals in other sports (triathlon, road cycling, etc.) and so on. And set interim goals, whether for pace, distance, weight loss, or anything else that will give you a regular opportunity during your longer training calendar to acknowledge your progress short of the 'ultimate' goal. Apart from planning, as soon as you set a goal you may see a change in your daily rowing.

Another tool you can use is well-known training information, such as that available on the Concept2 web sites (the British site is a favorite for many), the Canadian National Team web site, and Mike Caviston's Wolverine Plan. Does the information in these programs look like it would work for you? Do you see a component you like? Can you take anything from it to help you learn more about how to get your body functioning the way you want it to?

As you train to improve, whether or not it is to prepare you to compete in a race, incorporate both steady-state rowing and interval work. You will find more on these two basic approaches to exercise in other writings, including the appendices later in this book. Consider that each type of workout has multiple variables you can use. Intervals can be shorter or longer; and they can be based on the number of strokes rowed, elapsed time, breathing, heart rate and other parameters. Keep in mind that the intervals of rest are just as important as the intervals of harder work. A beginner can modify a racer's interval workout by extending the rest periods, for example, as well as by slowing the pace or reducing the power applied. Steady state pieces can also be either entirely comfortable or rowed as a challenge, such as trying to see how fast a pace you can maintain for the duration. So there is a wide variety of steady state work you can do not only because you can choose different distances and compare your reaction to using time rather than distance as your measure, but also because you can row a steady state piece at anything from an easy paddle to the fastest pace you can maintain.

Recognize that progress is incremental and use your log book to keep track of your progress. And remember that improvement may not occur every day and every week; the incremental steps may not all be "up." But you will make substantial progress over time. When training to race, your goal will be something that you simply cannot accomplish today. By creating progress incrementally, you can change your fitness/speed to such a degree that you will be able to perform at a level well beyond your present ability. And if you are not planning to race, you can still accomplish the same feat by training to improve. You will create a new normal for yourself.

Ron is accomplished at identifying and preparing for the races he most wants to win. He adjusts his training to reach his best preparation for each race. And throughout the year he is working on overall fitness, from building and maintaining his aerobic base to addressing perceived weaknesses based on last year's performance.

Mel can use improvement techniques as soon as she begins to exercise with any regularity. In fact, knowing that she can vary what she does may be the best tool she has to help her keep rowing. She does not have to repeat the same thing every day. She can take on a number of variations at her own speed. And it enables her to progress incrementally so that she avoids the trap of feeling her efforts are wasted.

Andie has long been a regular exerciser and is looking forward to making a difference in her routine and her performance. She has often wondered whether she is limited by her body type, sports history or current fitness. Using a new routine of steady state workouts and interval training shows her quickly that she is not as limited as she thought.

1

Date, day, time, location: _____

Feeling of energy/health before: _____*during:*_____ *after:* _____

Challenges: _____

Max effort/breathing/pulse: _____

Core: _____

Stretching: _____

Successes: _____

Other: _____

Time/Distance/Totals, if any: _____

2

Date, day, time, location: _____

Feeling of energy/health before: _____*during:*_____ *after:* _____

Challenges: _____

Max effort/breathing/pulse: _____

Core: _____

Stretching: _____

Successes: _____

Other: _____

Time/Distance/Totals, if any: _____

3

Date, day, time, location: _____

Feeling of energy/health before: _____*during:*_____ *after:* _____

Challenges: _____

Max effort/breathing/pulse: _____

Core: _____

Stretching: _____

Successes: _____

Other: _____

Time/Distance/Totals, if any: _____

4

Date, day, time, location: _____

Feeling of energy/health before: _____*during:*_____ *after:* _____

Challenges: _____

Max effort/breathing/pulse: _____

Core: _____

What shall I do today . . . heute . . . hoy . . . aujourd'hui . . . oggi . . . idag . . . tanaan . . . avui . . .

Stretching: _____

Successes: _____

Other: _____

Time/Distance/Totals, if any: _____

5

Date, day, time, location: _____

Feeling of energy/health before: _____during:_____ after: _____

Challenges: _____

Max effort/breathing/pulse: _____

Core: _____

Stretching: _____

Successes: _____

Other: _____

Time/Distance/Totals, if any: _____

6

Date, day, time, location: _____

Feeling of energy/health before: _____during:_____ after: _____

Challenges: _____

Max effort/breathing/pulse: _____

Core: _____

Stretching: _____

Successes: _____

Other: _____

Time/Distance/Totals, if any: _____

7

Date, day, time, location: _____

Feeling of energy/health before: _____during:_____ after: _____

Challenges: _____

Max effort/breathing/pulse: _____

Core: _____

Stretching: _____

Successes: _____

Other: _____

Time/Distance/Totals, if any: _____

8

Date, day, time, location: _____

Feeling of energy/health before: _____*during:*_____ *after:* _____

Challenges: _____

Max effort/breathing/pulse: _____

Core: _____

Stretching: _____

Successes: _____

Other: _____

Time/Distance/Totals, if any: _____

9

Date, day, time, location: _____

Feeling of energy/health before: _____*during:*_____ *after:* _____

Challenges: _____

Max effort/breathing/pulse: _____

Core: _____

Stretching: _____

Successes: _____

Other: _____

Time/Distance/Totals, if any: _____

10

Date, day, time, location: _____

Feeling of energy/health before: _____*during:*_____ *after:* _____

Challenges: _____

Max effort/breathing/pulse: _____

Core: _____

Stretching: _____

Successes: _____

Other: _____

Time/Distance/Totals, if any: _____

11

Date, day, time, location: _____

Feeling of energy/health before: _____*during:*_____ *after:* _____

Challenges: _____

Max effort/breathing/pulse: _____

Core: _____

Stretching: _____

Successes: _____

Other: _____

Time/Distance/Totals, if any: _____

12

Date, day, time, location: _____

Feeling of energy/health before: _____ *during:* _____ *after:* _____

Challenges: _____

Max effort/breathing/pulse: _____

Core: _____

Stretching: _____

Successes: _____

Other: _____

Time/Distance/Totals, if any: _____

13

Date, day, time, location: _____

Feeling of energy/health before: _____ *during:* _____ *after:* _____

Challenges: _____

Max effort/breathing/pulse: _____

Core: _____

Stretching: _____

Successes: _____

Other: _____

Time/Distance/Totals, if any: _____

14

Date, day, time, location: _____

Feeling of energy/health before: _____ *during:* _____ *after:* _____

Challenges: _____

Max effort/breathing/pulse: _____

Core: _____

Stretching: _____

Successes: _____

Other: _____

Time/Distance/Totals, if any: _____

15

Date, day, time, location: _____

Feeling of energy/health before: _____during:_____ after: _____

Challenges: _____

Max effort/breathing/pulse: _____

Core: _____

Stretching: _____

Successes: _____

Other: _____

Time/Distance/Totals, if any: _____

16

Date, day, time, location: _____

Feeling of energy/health before: _____during:_____ after: _____

Challenges: _____

Max effort/breathing/pulse: _____

Core: _____

Stretching: _____

Successes: _____

Other: _____

Time/Distance/Totals, if any: _____

17

Date, day, time, location: _____

Feeling of energy/health before: _____during:_____ after: _____

Challenges: _____ _____

Max effort/breathing/pulse: _____

Core: _____ _____

Stretching: _____

Successes: _____

Other: _____

Time/Distance/Totals, if any: _____

18

Date, day, time, location: _____

Feeling of energy/health before: _____during:_____ after: _____

Challenges: _____

Max effort/breathing/pulse: _____

Core: _____

Stretching: _____

Successes: _____

Other: _____

Time/Distance/Totals, if any: _____

19

Date, day, time, location: _____

Feeling of energy/health before: _____ *during:* _____ *after:* _____

Challenges: _____

Max effort/breathing/pulse: _____

Core: _____

Stretching: _____

Successes: _____

Other: _____

Time/Distance/Totals, if any: _____

20

Date, day, time, location: _____

Feeling of energy/health before: _____ *during:* _____ *after:* _____

Challenges: _____

Max effort/breathing/pulse: _____

Core: _____

Stretching: _____

Successes: _____

Other: _____

Time/Distance/Totals, if any: _____

21

Date, day, time, location: _____

Feeling of energy/health before: _____ *during:* _____ *after:* _____

Challenges: _____

Max effort/breathing/pulse: _____

Core: _____

Stretching: _____

Successes: _____

Other: _____

Time/Distance/Totals, if any: _____

22

Date, day, time, location: _____

Feeling of energy/health before: _____ *during:* _____ *after:* _____

Challenges: _____

Max effort/breathing/pulse: _____

Core: _____

Stretching: _____

Successes: _____

Other: _____

Time/Distance/Totals, if any: _____

23

Date, day, time, location: _____

Feeling of energy/health before: _____ *during:* _____ *after:* _____

Challenges: _____

Max effort/breathing/pulse: _____

Core: _____

Stretching: _____

Successes: _____

Other: _____

Time/Distance/Totals, if any: _____

24

Date, day, time, location: _____

Feeling of energy/health before: _____ *during:* _____ *after:* _____

Challenges: _____

Max effort/breathing/pulse: _____

Core: _____

Stretching: _____

Successes: _____

Other: _____

Time/Distance/Totals, if any: _____

25

Date, day, time, location: _____

Feeling of energy/health before: _____ *during:* _____ *after:* _____

Challenges: _____

Max effort/breathing/pulse: _____

Core: _____

What shall I do today . . . heute . . . hoy . . . aujourd'hui . . . oggi . . . idag . . . tanaan . . . avui . . .

Stretching: _____

Successes: _____

Other: _____

Time/Distance/Totals, if any: _____

26

Date, day, time, location: _____

Feeling of energy/health before: _____ during: _____ after: _____

Challenges: _____

Max effort/breathing/pulse: _____

Core: _____

Stretching: _____

Successes: _____

Other: _____

Time/Distance/Totals, if any: _____

27

Date, day, time, location: _____

Feeling of energy/health before: _____ during: _____ after: _____

Challenges: _____

Max effort/breathing/pulse: _____

Core: _____

Stretching: _____

Successes: _____

Other: _____

Time/Distance/Totals, if any: _____

28

Date, day, time, location: _____

Feeling of energy/health before: _____ during: _____ after: _____

Challenges: _____

Max effort/breathing/pulse: _____

Core: _____

Stretching: _____

Successes: _____

Other: _____

Time/Distance/Totals, if any: _____

29

Date, day, time, location: _____

Feeling of energy/health before: _____*during:*_____ *after:* _____

Challenges: _____

Max effort/breathing/pulse: _____

Core: _____

Stretching: _____

Successes: _____

Other: _____

Time/Distance/Totals, if any: _____

30

Date, day, time, location: _____

Feeling of energy/health before: _____*during:*_____ *after:* _____

Challenges: _____

Max effort/breathing/pulse: _____

Core: _____

Stretching: _____

Successes: _____

Other: _____

Time/Distance/Totals, if any: _____

31

Date, day, time, location: _____

Feeling of energy/health before: _____*during:*_____ *after:* _____

Challenges: _____

Max effort/breathing/pulse: _____

Core: _____

Stretching: _____

Successes: _____

Other: _____

Time/Distance/Totals, if any: _____

Extra Workouts 1

Date, day, time, location: _____

Feeling of energy/health before: _____ *during:* _____ *after:* _____

Challenges: _____

Max effort/breathing/pulse: _____

Core: _____

Stretching: _____

Successes: _____

Other: _____

Time/Distance/Totals, if any: _____

Extra 2

Date, day, time, location: _____

Feeling of energy/health before: _____ *during:* _____ *after:* _____

Challenges: _____

Max effort/breathing/pulse: _____

Core: _____

Stretching: _____

Successes: _____

Other: _____

Time/Distance/Totals, if any: _____

Extra 3

Date, day, time, location: _____

Feeling of energy/health before: _____ *during:* _____ *after:* _____

Challenges: _____

Max effort/breathing/pulse: _____

Core: _____

Stretching: _____

Successes: _____

Other: _____

Time/Distance/Totals, if any: _____

Extra 4

Date, day, time, location: _____

Feeling of energy/health before: _____ *during:* _____ *after:* _____

Challenges: _____

Max effort/breathing/pulse: _____

Core: _____

Stretching: _____

Successes: _____

Other: _____

Time/Distance/Totals, if any: _____

Extra 5

Date, day, time, location: _____

Feeling of energy/health before: _____during:_____ after: _____

Challenges: _____

Max effort/breathing/pulse: _____

Core: _____

Stretching: _____

Successes: _____

Other: _____

Time/Distance/Totals, if any: _____

End of Month Scoring

Method One: Basic (Number of days I exercised this month):_____
    Ultimate Goal: Every Day
    My Goal for This Month Was: _____
    My Goal for Next Month Is: _____
Method Two: Subtraction (Days I Rowed Minus Days Not):_____
    Initial Goal: Exceed Zero (row at least half the days)
    Ultimate Goal: Same as days in the month.
    My Goal for This Month Was: _____
    My Goal for Next Month Is: _____
Method Three: Division (Percentage = Days Rowed Divided by Total Days): _____
    Ultimate Goal: 100%
    My Goal for This Month Was:_____
    My Goal for Next Month Is: _____

Other Scores and Data for Month (Goals set and met; Times rowed; Distances rowed; Other):

_____

_____

_____

_____

_____

_____

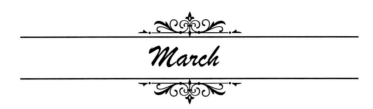

March

"A bear, however hard he tries,
grows tubby without exercise."
   A.A. Milne

"Nothing happens until something moves."
   Albert Einstein

"Use it or lose it."
   Jimmy Connors

"You don't get old from age, you get old from inactivity."
   Jack LaLanne

"The doctor of the future will give no medicine, but instead will interest his patients in the care of the human frame, in diet, and in the cause and prevention of disease."
   Thomas Edison

"Exercise may be the closest thing to the fountain of youth available. It improves overall health and appearance. It can maintain some of the body's functions that decline with aging. It can even restore some functions that have already declined."
   Merck, at 806

"When you sum up the powerful effects of moderate exercise on the health of older people, it's hard to imagine why we aren't all out there working up a sweat. . . . The goal is to exercise on a regular basis at least several days a week."
   Successful Aging, at 138

March – The Core: Use It; Rebuild It; Maintain It

When I began to train recently for a fall race (not having raced for a couple of years), I quickly realized that I needed to get my core back into shape. The standard condition of the muscles in and around the gut and lower back, collectively called the core, is abominable in most of us. At the time I began to train, I felt I was in decent shape. No question, I was in better shape than the average person. I was even doing some core exercises already as part of my routine, here and there, sometimes. And yet I had developed a small paunch that seemed to reflect not just the accumulation of some belly fat but also an absence of conditioning. And, worse yet, my core muscles were weakened, rarely used and very out of shape.

So what, you may ask, if some unnecessary muscles are out of shape? We do not all have to be body builders. We do not need, nor should we want, to have 'six-packs' of buff, visible abdominal muscle groups. But if you can overcome the natural reaction against seeking "the look" (which is not the point), you will have to agree that a fit, healthy set of core muscles is one of the keys to health and fitness. The core muscles, front, back and sides, help with posture, which helps with breathing. They protect our guts, where digestion and so many other organ functions critical to our health take place. And they help hold the back in place and reduce the likelihood of back aches and pains. Finally, training these muscles to be strong can provide the less obvious benefit that it also trains them to relax, which may well be just as critical a path to the goal of minimizing back pain.

Instead of just selecting one or two core exercises to do each day, plan out two or three months and make it your goal to get core-fit. Select a dozen or more varied core exercises that will work a range of the many muscles in and around the core of your body. Begin to do every one of them every day. You will probably not be able to do them all at one time when you first begin, at least not for a serious set of repetitions. That is fine; the goal is overall, long term gain, not whether you can prove yourself equal to some standard today. And you will almost certainly have some very sore muscles if you overdo core work early on. So here is a suggestion for becoming serious about the core in a moderate way:

- Compile a list of a dozen or more core exercises.
- Start by doing at least one rep of every exercise in the set each day.
- Think of it as becoming familiar with how to do them and the order in which you want to proceed with them.
- Consider alternating between muscles deep and on the surface, muscles on the front and on the back and on the side, exercises that are dynamic and those that are static.
- Get through the whole set of exercises each day, even if you do very few of each as if only to remind yourself of the positioning for each core exercise.

- Then, each day you proceed, gradually increase the number of repetitions of each exercise and/or the duration of each repetition if holding a position is involved.
- Each week and month consider the progress you have made.
- Enjoy the feeling of being able to do more without a feeling of weakness or pain.

This approach can allow you to minimize muscle soreness on a daily basis while you make substantial progress over a period of weeks.

To further develop core fitness and to maintain what you achieve, continue to set goals and expectations after you complete the initial three months. Assuming you have achieved a basic level of competence with a full set of core exercises (such as 10 reps of each with reasonably-timed holds), do one or more of the following to maintain and build on that progress:

- Make the full set part of your daily workout;
- Add or substitute one or more entirely different core exercises for part of the set;
- Take a core training class such as Pilates or what some gyms call basic training or boot camp; and
- Increase the time and/or reps of one or more of your standard set, and alternate which ones you emphasize week by week.

Ron has been competing for many years. As he aged through his 40s and 50s, he learned that he had to do more work just to maintain his basic fitness, much less get in shape for the peak fitness he wanted for race day. He might have thought of a trim waist and fit core as automatic results of his general exercise regimen when he was in his 30s, but no longer. He has added exercises to his routine repeatedly and takes them more seriously as his body has tended to become weaker every year he has aged. One of the areas of exercise he redoubled his efforts on was working the core.

Mel had never done sit-ups or other core exercises since her gym classes in school. She began a pre-set routine and quickly found her gut so sore that she swore off the exercises for a week until Andie explained how she could work up to a routine gently. Then she set out to break her body's muscles into the routine gradually, more comfortably – and more successfully.

Andie had done many core exercises in a variety of classes but had never included them outside of classes as part of her regular exercise. Now she heard the message about the importance of the core. She hoped that getting her core more fit would make it easier for her to develop greater overall fitness. So, slowly at first, she started spending about ten minutes on her core every day after her other exercise. One month into the new routine, she saw progress. And she liked what she saw and felt.

What shall I do today . . . heute . . . hoy . . . aujourd'hui . . . oggi . . . idag . . . tanaan . . . avui . . .

1

Date, day, time, location: _____

Feeling of energy/health before: _____ *during:* _____ *after:* _____

Challenges: _____

Max effort/breathing/pulse: _____

Core: _____

Stretching: _____

Successes: _____

Other: _____

Time/Distance/Totals, if any: _____

2

Date, day, time, location: _____

Feeling of energy/health before: _____ *during:* _____ *after:* _____

Challenges: _____

Max effort/breathing/pulse: _____

Core: _____

Stretching: _____

Successes: _____

Other: _____

Time/Distance/Totals, if any: _____

3

Date, day, time, location: _____

Feeling of energy/health before: _____ *during:* _____ *after:* _____

Challenges: _____

Max effort/breathing/pulse: _____

Core: _____

Stretching: _____

Successes: _____

Other: _____

Time/Distance/Totals, if any: _____

4

Date, day, time, location: _____

Feeling of energy/health before: _____ *during:* _____ *after:* _____

Challenges: _____

Max effort/breathing/pulse: _____

Core: _____

Stretching: _____

Successes: _____

Other: _____

Time/Distance/Totals, if any: _____

5

Date, day, time, location: _____

Feeling of energy/health before: _____ *during:* _____ *after:* _____

Challenges: _____

Max effort/breathing/pulse: _____

Core: _____

Stretching: _____

Successes: _____

Other: _____

Time/Distance/Totals, if any: _____

6

Date, day, time, location: _____

Feeling of energy/health before: _____ *during:* _____ *after:* _____

Challenges: _____

Max effort/breathing/pulse: _____

Core: _____

Stretching: _____

Successes: _____

Other: _____

Time/Distance/Totals, if any: _____

7

Date, day, time, location: _____

Feeling of energy/health before: _____ *during:* _____ *after:* _____

Challenges: _____

Max effort/breathing/pulse: _____

Core: _____

Stretching: _____

Successes: _____

Other: _____

Time/Distance/Totals, if any: _____

8

Date, day, time, location: _____

Feeling of energy/health before: _____*during:*_____ *after:* _____

Challenges: _____

Max effort/breathing/pulse: _____

Core: _____

Stretching: _____

Successes: _____

Other: _____

Time/Distance/Totals, if any: _____

9

Date, day, time, location: _____

Feeling of energy/health before: _____*during:*_____ *after:* _____

Challenges: _____

Max effort/breathing/pulse: _____

Core: _____

Stretching: _____

Successes: _____

Other: _____

Time/Distance/Totals, if any: _____

10

Date, day, time, location: _____

Feeling of energy/health before: _____*during:*_____ *after:* _____

Challenges: _____

Max effort/breathing/pulse: _____

Core: _____

Stretching: _____

Successes: _____

Other: _____

Time/Distance/Totals, if any: _____

11

Date, day, time, location: _____

Feeling of energy/health before: _____*during:*_____ *after:* _____

Challenges: _____

Max effort/breathing/pulse: _____

Core: _____

Stretching: _____

Successes: _____

Other: _____

Time/Distance/Totals, if any: _____

12

Date, day, time, location: _____

Feeling of energy/health before: _____*during:*_____ *after:* _____

Challenges: _____

Max effort/breathing/pulse: _____

Core: _____

Stretching: _____

Successes: _____

Other: _____

Time/Distance/Totals, if any: _____

13

Date, day, time, location: _____

Feeling of energy/health before: _____*during:*_____ *after:* _____

Challenges: _____

Max effort/breathing/pulse: _____

Core: _____

Stretching: _____

Successes: _____

Other: _____

Time/Distance/Totals, if any: _____

14

Date, day, time, location: _____

Feeling of energy/health before: _____*during:*_____ *after:* _____

Challenges: _____

Max effort/breathing/pulse: _____

Core: _____

Stretching: _____

Successes: _____

Other: _____

Time/Distance/Totals, if any: _____

15

Date, day, time, location: _____
Feeling of energy/health before: _____ *during:* _____ *after:* _____
Challenges: _____
Max effort/breathing/pulse: _____
Core: _____
Stretching: _____
Successes: _____
Other: _____
Time/Distance/Totals, if any: _____

16

Date, day, time, location: _____
Feeling of energy/health before: _____ *during:* _____ *after:* _____
Challenges: _____
Max effort/breathing/pulse: _____
Core: _____
Stretching: _____
Successes: _____
Other: _____
Time/Distance/Totals, if any: _____

17

Date, day, time, location: _____
Feeling of energy/health before: _____ *during:* _____ *after:* _____
Challenges: _____
Max effort/breathing/pulse: _____
Core: _____
Stretching: _____
Successes: _____
Other: _____
Time/Distance/Totals, if any: _____

18

Date, day, time, location: _____
Feeling of energy/health before: _____ *during:* _____ *after:* _____
Challenges: _____
Max effort/breathing/pulse: _____
Core: _____

Stretching: _____

Successes: _____

Other: _____

Time/Distance/Totals, if any: _____

19

Date, day, time, location: _____

Feeling of energy/health before: _____ *during:* _____ *after:* _____

Challenges: _____

Max effort/breathing/pulse: _____

Core: _____

Stretching: _____

Successes: _____

Other: _____

Time/Distance/Totals, if any: _____

20

Date, day, time, location: _____

Feeling of energy/health before: _____ *during:* _____ *after:* _____

Challenges: _____

Max effort/breathing/pulse: _____

Core: _____

Stretching: _____

Successes: _____

Other: _____

Time/Distance/Totals, if any: _____

21

Date, day, time, location: _____

Feeling of energy/health before: _____ *during:* _____ *after:* _____

Challenges: _____

Max effort/breathing/pulse: _____

Core: _____

Stretching: _____

Successes: _____

Other: _____

Time/Distance/Totals, if any: _____

22

Date, day, time, location: _____

Feeling of energy/health before: _____ *during:* _____ *after:* _____

Challenges: _____

Max effort/breathing/pulse: _____

Core: _____

Stretching: _____

Successes: _____

Other: _____

Time/Distance/Totals, if any: _____

23

Date, day, time, location: _____

Feeling of energy/health before: _____ *during:* _____ *after:* _____

Challenges: _____

Max effort/breathing/pulse: _____

Core: _____

Stretching: _____

Successes: _____

Other: _____

Time/Distance/Totals, if any: _____

24

Date, day, time, location: _____

Feeling of energy/health before: _____ *during:* _____ *after:* _____

Challenges: _____

Max effort/breathing/pulse: _____

Core: _____

Stretching: _____

Successes: _____

Other: _____

Time/Distance/Totals, if any: _____

25

Date, day, time, location: _____

Feeling of energy/health before: _____ *during:* _____ *after:* _____

Challenges: _____

Max effort/breathing/pulse: _____

Core: _____

Stretching: _____

Successes: _____

Other: _____

Time/Distance/Totals, if any: _____

26

Date, day, time, location: _____

Feeling of energy/health before: _____*during:*_____ *after:* _____

Challenges: _____

Max effort/breathing/pulse: _____

Core: _____

Stretching: _____

Successes: _____

Other: _____

Time/Distance/Totals, if any: _____

27

Date, day, time, location: _____

Feeling of energy/health before: _____*during:*_____ *after:* _____

Challenges: _____

Max effort/breathing/pulse: _____

Core: _____

Stretching: _____

Successes: _____

Other: _____

Time/Distance/Totals, if any: _____

28

Date, day, time, location: _____

Feeling of energy/health before: _____*during:*_____ *after:* _____

Challenges: _____

Max effort/breathing/pulse: _____

Core: _____

Stretching: _____

Successes: _____

Other: _____

Time/Distance/Totals, if any: _____

29
Date, day, time, location: _____
Feeling of energy/health before: _____ *during:* _____ *after:* _____
Challenges: _____
Max effort/breathing/pulse: _____
Core: _____
Stretching: _____
Successes: _____
Other: _____
Time/Distance/Totals, if any: _____

30
Date, day, time, location: _____
Feeling of energy/health before: _____ *during:* _____ *after:* _____
Challenges: _____
Max effort/breathing/pulse: _____
Core: _____
Stretching: _____
Successes: _____
Other: _____
Time/Distance/Totals, if any: _____

31
Date, day, time, location: _____
Feeling of energy/health before: _____ *during:* _____ *after:* _____
Challenges: _____
Max effort/breathing/pulse: _____
Core: _____
Stretching: _____
Successes: _____
Other: _____
Time/Distance/Totals, if any: _____

Extra Workouts 1

Date, day, time, location: _____

Feeling of energy/health before: _____during:_____ after: _____

Challenges: _____

Max effort/breathing/pulse: _____

Core: _____

Stretching: _____

Successes: _____

Other: _____

Time/Distance/Totals, if any: _____

Extra 2

Date, day, time, location: _____

Feeling of energy/health before: _____during:_____ after: _____

Challenges: _____

Max effort/breathing/pulse: _____

Core: _____

Stretching: _____

Successes: _____

Other: _____

Time/Distance/Totals, if any: _____

Extra 3

Date, day, time, location: _____

Feeling of energy/health before: _____during:_____ after: _____

Challenges: _____

Max effort/breathing/pulse: _____

Core: _____

Stretching: _____

Successes: _____

Other: _____

Time/Distance/Totals, if any: _____

Extra 4

Date, day, time, location: _____

Feeling of energy/health before: _____during:_____ after: _____

Challenges: _____

Max effort/breathing/pulse: _____

Core: _____

What shall I do today . . . heute . . . hoy . . . aujourd'hui . . . oggi . . . idag . . . tanaan . . . avui . . .

Stretching: _____

Successes: _____

Other: _____

Time/Distance/Totals, if any: _____

Extra 5

Date, day, time, location: _____

Feeling of energy/health before: _____ *during:* _____ *after:* _____

Challenges: _____

Max effort/breathing/pulse: _____

Core: _____

Stretching: _____

Successes: _____

Other: _____

Time/Distance/Totals, if any: _____

End of Month Scoring

Method One: Basic (Number of days I exercised this month):_____
    Ultimate Goal: Every Day
    My Goal for This Month Was: _____
    My Goal for Next Month Is: _____
Method Two: Subtraction (Days I Rowed Minus Days Not):_____
    Initial Goal: Exceed Zero (row at least half the days)
    Ultimate Goal: Same as days in the month.
    My Goal for This Month Was: _____
    My Goal for Next Month Is: _____
Method Three: Division (Percentage = Days Rowed Divided by Total Days): _____
    Ultimate Goal: 100%
    My Goal for This Month Was:_____
    My Goal for Next Month Is: _____

Other Scores and Data for Month (Goals set and met; Times rowed; Distances rowed; Other):

_____

_____

_____

_____

_____

_____

_____

Season Recap and Change

<u>Scoring</u>

You have calculated your score at the end of each month. Take a season-long look at your progress. Where have you improved during the three months of this season? Compare season to season as the year progresses. Most importantly, once you calculate your score, consider whether it correlates with how you feel.

_____

_____

_____

_____

_____

<u>Goals Accomplished</u>

Look back on your goals for the past season. Did you set goals based on how many days you rowed? Did you set goals to row longer or harder each day? If you are succeeding with both of those challenges, how are you doing at including core work and stretching each day? (Are you keeping track of that?) Do you also set goals for distances rowed or pace? Have you planned to take a rowing class or attend a rowing event? For these and other goals you may have set three months ago, look back and record here how you did.

_____

_____

_____

_____

_____

_____

Goals Looking Ahead

Once you have looked back, plan ahead. Set some goals. Make them realistic based on your past experience, events coming up and your other plans for the coming three months.

_____

_____

_____

_____

_____

Changes for Variety

Do you cross-train for variety? How can you modify that in the coming season? Plan a vacation based on doing something active you would enjoy. Add an aerobics or spinning or pilates class or some weight lifting or yoga or something else you may not normally do.

_____

_____

_____

_____

_____

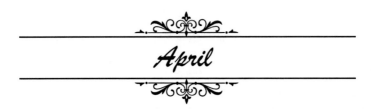

April

"He who enjoys good health is rich, though he knows it not."
  Italian proverb

"If you're tired and pooped out all the time, do you have love and compassion in your heart for your fellow man? You don't even like yourself!"
  Jack LaLanne

"Older age is not a reason to stop exercising. And it should not stop people from starting. In fact, doing regular exercise becomes more important as people age. Exercise can help keep older people active and living independently longer. Exercise can make even the frailest older person stronger and more fit."
  Merck, at 805

"As recently as the 1960s, many people believed that the elderly should curtail their activity because exercise could be hazardous to their health."
  Encyclopedia, at 583

"Exercise and temperance can preserve something of our early strength even in old age."
  Cicero

"See what daily exercise does for one."
  Seneca (4 BC to 65 AD)

"[V]ery old people – even those who have never exercised before – are capable of becoming more physically fit. . . . Even as time conspires to rob us of our physical strength, balance, and endurance, we can fight the clock. And many older people are winning that fight."
  Successful Aging, at 139

April – Cross-Train to Supplement Your Rowing

Some people naturally use cross-training for fitness because they engage in multiple sports for recreation. Rowers and bicyclists may cross-country ski in the winter, for example. Basketball and football players may row for the stamina and leg strength it gives them. Participants in many sports lift weights to strengthen the muscle groups that are key to their sports, as well as to work the complementary muscle groups that help balance the body. Many athletes use yoga for flexibility, strength and whole-body coordination.

If you decide to use cross-training to work toward a race, plan it out accordingly. For example, it may make sense to begin your cross-training three months to a year before the target event. If you want to cycle to improve your aerobic base, for example, start months in advance. The benefits will not accrue overnight. If you intend to lift weights to build up your strength, start early enough to be able to use those stronger muscles in your aerobic work. Plan to taper off well before your race.

If you are rowing not to race but for health and fitness, consider what cross-training you might want to try and when it will fit your schedule. If your program is designed for your general health and fitness rather than for a particular event or deadline, you can sample and use cross-training at any time. Make it part of your regular routine or mix it into and out of your routine. If you do not have an impending deadline but the seasons are changing, try something new just for the challenge and variety. I suggest, however, that you keep your basic routine intact as much as you can, as well. In other words, if you start playing soccer, do not stop rowing altogether. If you begin to lift weights, do it as a second workout to your rowing or alternate days with rowing. If you want to add core work or yoga, make it part of your weekly schedule along with rowing.

Some suggestions:

- Use restraint: Do not start something new like a weekend warrior, going at it as if you were ready to go all out. Avoid injury and unnecessary soreness. It is amazing how out of shape some muscles can be despite our other, general physical activity. Getting sore does not mean you hurt yourself, but it may mean you overdid it. More importantly, excessive soreness can be discouraging. The best response to that is to keep at it, but more moderately. The best solution to the issue of excessive soreness is avoidance, not of the exercises but of the excess: Start easily and build gradually.
- Try something new: Our muscles are best trained for our usual activities. Try something that uses different muscles. Try something that sounds appealing because it is new.
- Do something you enjoy: Whether playing a sport or simply taking a walk, spending time moving doing something you enjoy will make it easier for you to continue the activity.

- Use cross-training to get stronger: Our muscles have not only the capacity but the natural tendency to diminish in strength as we age. That effect is dramatically speeded up with inactivity. Happily, the opposite is also true and, with regular activity, our muscles naturally will become stronger. Add something to your routine to build your strength.
- Add something different while still rowing to get in double workouts; increase the amount of exercise you get with something new instead of just more of the same. Bored with your routine? Try something else in addition and see how it changes the way your regular rowing feels.
- Use cross-training to mark and enjoy the changing seasons: There are so many ways to use the changing seasons to add to your exercise. If you are in a colder climate, you will enjoy getting outside more once it warms up, whether with cycling, tennis, swimming, or any of many other activities. But also, when it gets colder, try indoor options like a spinning class, swimming in the pool, and tennis at the health club. And try skiing, snow-shoeing or other outdoor cold-weather activities.
- Look for your weaknesses and work on those: Do you hate to do push-ups? Then try them for a week. (Remember, you can find a way to start them easily; then use your daily routine to build up your capacity and strength.) Cannot do a pull-up? Work on them for a month. Feeling weak on the drive when rowing? Try two or three weight lifting exercises to strengthen the quads.

Ron's training focuses primarily on rowing; his goal is to row fast during the small number of key races that matter most to him. But he learned long ago that judicious use of cross-training would enhance his performance. Weight lifting is a regular part of his routine. One of his favorite cross-training exercises is using his road bike, where he can work his legs and wind with less overall demand on his body. Older experienced competitors like Ron have a wealth of information that may not apply directly to a novice's routine but can provide insights and ideas for cross-training that you can use to enrich your rowing.

Mel's first reactions to the suggestion to cross-train were that she was already doing more than ever before — and she wasn't "training" so that it would be a mistake to change. But once she tried a couple of different exercises besides rowing she quickly caught on that it helped her improve faster and feel a greater sense of satisfaction.

Andie was used to doing many different forms of exercise, but usually only one at a time. She would focus on yoga for a few months. Then she might try Pilates or kick-boxing lessons. Now she made rowing the centerpiece of her program and added other classes or activities in a loose rotation to supplement that. And, for the first time, she began to select activities based on how they helped her performance.

1

Date, day, time, location: _____

Feeling of energy/health before: _____*during:*_____ *after:* _____

Challenges: _____

Max effort/breathing/pulse: _____

Core: _____

Stretching: _____

Successes: _____

Other: _____

Time/Distance/Totals, if any: _____

2

Date, day, time, location: _____

Feeling of energy/health before: _____*during:*_____ *after:* _____

Challenges: _____

Max effort/breathing/pulse: _____

Core: _____

Stretching: _____

Successes: _____

Other: _____

Time/Distance/Totals, if any: _____

3

Date, day, time, location: _____

Feeling of energy/health before: _____*during:*_____ *after:* _____

Challenges: _____

Max effort/breathing/pulse: _____

Core: _____

Stretching: _____

Successes: _____

Other: _____

Time/Distance/Totals, if any: _____

4

Date, day, time, location: _____

Feeling of energy/health before: _____*during:*_____ *after:* _____

Challenges: _____

Max effort/breathing/pulse: _____

Core: _____

What shall I do today . . . heute . . . hoy . . . aujourd'hui . . . oggi . . . idag . . . tanaan . . . avui . . .

Stretching: _____

Successes: _____

Other: _____

Time/Distance/Totals, if any: _____

5

Date, day, time, location: _____

Feeling of energy/health before: _____ *during:* _____ *after:* _____

Challenges: _____

Max effort/breathing/pulse: _____

Core: _____

Stretching: _____

Successes: _____

Other: _____

Time/Distance/Totals, if any: _____

6

Date, day, time, location: _____

Feeling of energy/health before: _____ *during:* _____ *after:* _____

Challenges: _____

Max effort/breathing/pulse: _____

Core: _____

Stretching: _____

Successes: _____

Other: _____

Time/Distance/Totals, if any: _____

7

Date, day, time, location: _____

Feeling of energy/health before: _____ *during:* _____ *after:* _____

Challenges: _____

Max effort/breathing/pulse: _____

Core: _____

Stretching: _____

Successes: _____

Other: _____

Time/Distance/Totals, if any: _____

8

Date, day, time, location: _____

Feeling of energy/health before: _____*during:*_____ *after:* _____

Challenges: _____

Max effort/breathing/pulse: _____

Core: _____

Stretching: _____

Successes: _____

Other: _____

Time/Distance/Totals, if any: _____

9

Date, day, time, location: _____

Feeling of energy/health before: _____*during:*_____ *after:* _____

Challenges: _____

Max effort/breathing/pulse: _____

Core: _____

Stretching: _____

Successes: _____

Other: _____

Time/Distance/Totals, if any: _____

10

Date, day, time, location: _____

Feeling of energy/health before: _____*during:*_____ *after:* _____

Challenges: _____

Max effort/breathing/pulse: _____

Core: _____

Stretching: _____

Successes: _____

Other: _____

Time/Distance/Totals, if any: _____

11

Date, day, time, location: _____

Feeling of energy/health before: _____*during:*_____ *after:* _____

Challenges: _____

Max effort/breathing/pulse: _____

Core: _____

What shall I do today . . . heute . . . hoy . . . aujourd'hui . . . oggi . . . idag . . . tanaan . . . avui . . .

Stretching: _____

Successes: _____

Other: _____

Time/Distance/Totals, if any: _____

12

Date, day, time, location: _____

Feeling of energy/health before: _____*during:*_____ *after:* _____

Challenges: _____

Max effort/breathing/pulse: _____

Core: _____

Stretching: _____

Successes: _____

Other: _____

Time/Distance/Totals, if any: _____

13

Date, day, time, location: _____

Feeling of energy/health before: _____*during:*_____ *after:* _____

Challenges: _____

Max effort/breathing/pulse: _____

Core: _____

Stretching: _____

Successes: _____

Other: _____

Time/Distance/Totals, if any: _____

14

Date, day, time, location: _____

Feeling of energy/health before: _____*during:*_____ *after:* _____

Challenges: _____

Max effort/breathing/pulse: _____

Core: _____

Stretching: _____

Successes: _____

Other: _____

Time/Distance/Totals, if any: _____

15

Date, day, time, location: _____

Feeling of energy/health before: _____ *during:* _____ *after:* _____

Challenges: _____

Max effort/breathing/pulse: _____

Core: _____

Stretching: _____

Successes: _____

Other: _____

Time/Distance/Totals, if any: _____

16

Date, day, time, location: _____

Feeling of energy/health before: _____ *during:* _____ *after:* _____

Challenges: _____

Max effort/breathing/pulse: _____

Core: _____

Stretching: _____

Successes: _____

Other: _____

Time/Distance/Totals, if any: _____

17

Date, day, time, location: _____

Feeling of energy/health before: _____ *during:* _____ *after:* _____

Challenges: _____

Max effort/breathing/pulse: _____

Core: _____

Stretching: _____

Successes: _____

Other: _____

Time/Distance/Totals, if any: _____

18

Date, day, time, location: _____

Feeling of energy/health before: _____ *during:* _____ *after:* _____

Challenges: _____

Max effort/breathing/pulse: _____

Core: _____

What shall I do today . . . heute . . . hoy . . . aujourd'hui . . . oggi . . . idag . . . tanaan . . . avui . . .

Stretching: _____
Successes: _____
Other: _____
Time/Distance/Totals, if any: _____

19

Date, day, time, location: _____
Feeling of energy/health before: _____ *during:* _____ *after:* _____
Challenges: _____
Max effort/breathing/pulse: _____
Core: _____
Stretching: _____
Successes: _____
Other: _____
Time/Distance/Totals, if any: _____

20

Date, day, time, location: _____
Feeling of energy/health before: _____ *during:* _____ *after:* _____
Challenges: _____
Max effort/breathing/pulse: _____
Core: _____
Stretching: _____
Successes: _____
Other: _____
Time/Distance/Totals, if any: _____

21

Date, day, time, location: _____
Feeling of energy/health before: _____ *during:* _____ *after:* _____
Challenges: _____
Max effort/breathing/pulse: _____
Core: _____
Stretching: _____
Successes: _____
Other: _____
Time/Distance/Totals, if any: _____

22

Date, day, time, location: _____
Feeling of energy/health before: _____during:_____ after: _____
Challenges: _____
Max effort/breathing/pulse: _____
Core: _____
Stretching: _____
Successes: _____
Other: _____
Time/Distance/Totals, if any: _____

23

Date, day, time, location: _____
Feeling of energy/health before: _____during:_____ after: _____
Challenges: _____
Max effort/breathing/pulse: _____
Core: _____
Stretching: _____
Successes: _____
Other: _____
Time/Distance/Totals, if any: _____

24

Date, day, time, location: _____
Feeling of energy/health before: _____during:_____ after: _____
Challenges: _____
Max effort/breathing/pulse: _____
Core: _____
Stretching: _____
Successes: _____
Other: _____
Time/Distance/Totals, if any: _____

25

Date, day, time, location: _____
Feeling of energy/health before: _____during:_____ after: _____
Challenges: _____
Max effort/breathing/pulse: _____
Core: _____

Stretching: _____

Successes: _____

Other: _____

Time/Distance/Totals, if any: _____

26

Date, day, time, location: _____

Feeling of energy/health before: _____ *during:* _____ *after:* _____

Challenges: _____

Max effort/breathing/pulse: _____

Core: _____

Stretching: _____

Successes: _____

Other: _____

Time/Distance/Totals, if any: _____

27

Date, day, time, location: _____

Feeling of energy/health before: _____ *during:* _____ *after:* _____

Challenges: _____

Max effort/breathing/pulse: _____

Core: _____

Stretching: _____

Successes: _____

Other: _____

Time/Distance/Totals, if any: _____

28

Date, day, time, location: _____

Feeling of energy/health before: _____ *during:* _____ *after:* _____

Challenges: _____

Max effort/breathing/pulse: _____

Core: _____

Stretching: _____

Successes: _____

Other: _____

Time/Distance/Totals, if any: _____

29

Date, day, time, location: _____

Feeling of energy/health before: _____during:_____ after: _____

Challenges: _____

Max effort/breathing/pulse: _____

Core: _____

Stretching: _____

Successes: _____

Other: _____

Time/Distance/Totals, if any: _____

30

Date, day, time, location: _____

Feeling of energy/health before: _____during:_____ after: _____

Challenges: _____

Max effort/breathing/pulse: _____

Core: _____

Stretching: _____

Successes: _____

Other: _____

Time/Distance/Totals, if any: _____

31

Date, day, time, location: _____

Feeling of energy/health before: _____during:_____ after: _____

Challenges: _____

Max effort/breathing/pulse: _____

Core: _____

Stretching: _____

Successes: _____

Other: _____

Time/Distance/Totals, if any: _____

What shall I do today . . . heute . . . hoy . . . aujourd'hui . . . oggi . . . idag . . . tanaan . . . avui . . .

Extra Workouts 1
Date, day, time, location: _____
Feeling of energy/health before: _____during:_____ after: _____
Challenges: _____
Max effort/breathing/pulse: _____
Core: _____
Stretching: _____
Successes: _____
Other: _____
Time/Distance/Totals, if any: _____

Extra 2
Date, day, time, location: _____
Feeling of energy/health before: _____during:_____ after: _____
Challenges: _____
Max effort/breathing/pulse: _____
Core: _____
Stretching: _____
Successes: _____
Other: _____
Time/Distance/Totals, if any: _____

Extra 3
Date, day, time, location: _____
Feeling of energy/health before: _____during:_____ after: _____
Challenges: _____
Max effort/breathing/pulse: _____
Core: _____
Stretching: _____
Successes: _____
Other: _____
Time/Distance/Totals, if any: _____

Extra 4
Date, day, time, location: _____
Feeling of energy/health before: _____during:_____ after: _____
Challenges: _____
Max effort/breathing/pulse: _____
Core: _____

Stretching: _____

Successes: _____

Other: _____

Time/Distance/Totals, if any: _____

Extra 5

Date, day, time, location: _____

Feeling of energy/health before: _____ *during:* _____ *after:* _____

Challenges: _____

Max effort/breathing/pulse: _____

Core: _____

Stretching: _____

Successes: _____

Other: _____

Time/Distance/Totals, if any: _____

What shall I do today . . . heute . . . hoy . . . aujourd'hui . . . oggi . . . idag . . . tanaan . . . avui . . .

End of Month Scoring

Method One: Basic (Number of days I exercised this month):_____
    Ultimate Goal: Every Day
    My Goal for This Month Was: _____
    My Goal for Next Month Is: _____
Method Two: Subtraction (Days I Rowed Minus Days Not):_____
    Initial Goal: Exceed Zero (row at least half the days)
    Ultimate Goal: Same as days in the month.
    My Goal for This Month Was: _____
    My Goal for Next Month Is: _____
Method Three: Division (Percentage = Days Rowed Divided by Total Days): _____
    Ultimate Goal: 100%
    My Goal for This Month Was:_____
    My Goal for Next Month Is: _____

Other Scores and Data for Month (Goals set and met; Times rowed; Distances rowed; Other):

_____

_____

_____

_____

_____

_____

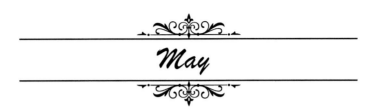

May

"*Physical activity and exercise can play an important role in preventing obesity, high blood pressure, heart disease, stroke, diabetes, some types of cancer, and other health problems, including such vexing problems as constipation. The best routine includes moderate physical activity for 30 minutes or more on all or most days of the week.*"
    Merck, at 30

"*How hard, how long, and how often to exercise are common questions. Starting with relatively less vigorous exercise for relatively short times is safest. How vigorous exercise is (intensity) can be determined . . . by observing how heavy breathing and sweating are. The intensity and length of exercise should be comfortable. Exercise is too intense if a person cannot comfortably talk.*"
    Merck, at 808

"*Regular physical activity may reverse the decline in the speed of nerve conduction that accompanies aging . . . .*"
    Encyclopedia, at 587

"*Even when all is known, the care of a man is not yet complete, because eating alone will not keep a man well; he must also take exercise. For food and exercise, while possessing opposite qualities, yet work together to produce health.*"
    Hippocrates

"*Better to hunt in fields, for health unbought,*
Than fee the doctor for a nauseous draught,
The Wise, for cure, on exercise depend;
God never made his work for man to mend."
    John Dryden

"*The frailty of old age is largely reversible. Most older people, even the very old and weak, have the capacity to remarkably increase their muscle strength, balance, walking ability, and overall aerobic power . . . . The key is to exercise regularly . . . .*"
    Successful Aging, at 143

May – Double Workouts

Exercising twice a day is not just for the extreme competitor. While two full-length, intense workouts in one day might be a rare event even for the coach-trained rowing team, there are ways anyone can use double workouts to enhance your health and fitness.

Perhaps the simplest begins with some methods of cross-training. You row each day and then add a yoga class or Pilates class three nights a week. On those days when you have a class in addition to rowing, you are doing double workouts. You will see benefits because you will gain the additional fitness the class offers while maintaining your rowing.

Another reason to use double workouts is to help you improve at the beginning of your training, when you feel like you cannot stay on the erg to row for long. You find you want to get up and quit after ten minutes, for example. One way to accept that and yet improve and eventually get past it is to get back on the erg a second time later in the day. It is a good scheduling exercise and you will find that several days of short double workouts will result in a day when you find you are perfectly OK with staying on the erg for a longer period during one exercise session. The duration of the second workout may not be directly additive, but it will increase your improvement compared to doing only one row a day. And once you lengthen your primary daily row you can use other exercises for your occasional second daily workout.

A third reason to use a second workout that does not involve pushing your limits is for recovery. If you feel you are rowing hard and become sore and tired, try a second easy row later in the day. Getting the blood flowing again can help with the speed and completeness of your physiological recovery from the earlier, more intense workout. So, for example, if you did a set of demanding two-minute pieces in the morning, try a 20-30 minute row at a slower pace later in the day. See how you feel the next day when you try your next challenging workout. You will find the "easy" row helps speed your recovery.

Let's return to using double workouts to do cross-training. If you decide you can benefit from lifting weights, insert it into your routine but do not give up your rowing, at least not every day you lift weights. At a minimum, you can use a later, easy row as noted above for faster recovery. And if your goal is to be faster sooner, you can complement the strength training with aerobic training later in the day. Just exercise judgment so that you get plenty of rest, good diet, and acknowledge that, if there comes a time when your muscles are not recovering adequately, that is a sign that you need a break that is different from a recovery row.

And that brings us to what may seem less like two workouts than a workout and a rest. Use the second workout exclusively for stretching. Relaxed yoga and other full-body stretching work that does not challenge your tired muscles in the same way as rowing does, but which helps increase your overall fitness, can be restful and productive at the same time.

Simply put, there are many ways to use double workouts to help you get more out of what you are doing. You may find that, like cross-training, this is a great topic to discuss with others you know who row. Experiment with what works for you.

Ron works out twice a day judiciously (off and on) throughout the year. He usually has a goal for each workout and sometimes can work at two goals in a day. After long years of training and competing, he has become sensitive to the limits to which he can push his body and what recovery it needs. And, as he ages, he is learning he has to change some of those routines to become faster even as he combats the weakening effects of aging.

Mel tried rowing twice a day after a discouraging two weeks of feeling she had reached a plateau as to how long she was willing to row. She quickly found after only a few days that she could translate her twice-a-day rows into one longer and harder row that she actually enjoyed. What had seemed interminable became easier and more productive.

Andie decided to add cross-training with rowing instead of replacing it, resulting in doing double workouts. One of her favorites was a boot camp class at the gym. The first time she got back on the rowing machine she felt very sore. But she quickly found that the boot camp exercises strengthened her rowing and her rowing helped her recover from the boot camp soreness and do better during the next class.

1

Date, day, time, location: _____

Feeling of energy/health before: _____ *during:* _____ *after:* _____

Challenges: _____

Max effort/breathing/pulse: _____

Core: _____

Stretching: _____

Successes: _____

Other: _____

Time/Distance/Totals, if any: _____

2

Date, day, time, location: _____

Feeling of energy/health before: _____ *during:* _____ *after:* _____

Challenges: _____

Max effort/breathing/pulse: _____

Core: _____

Stretching: _____

Successes: _____

Other: _____

Time/Distance/Totals, if any: _____

3

Date, day, time, location: _____

Feeling of energy/health before: _____ *during:* _____ *after:* _____

Challenges: _____

Max effort/breathing/pulse: _____

Core: _____

Stretching: _____

Successes: _____

Other: _____

Time/Distance/Totals, if any: _____

4

Date, day, time, location: _____

Feeling of energy/health before: _____ *during:* _____ *after:* _____

Challenges: _____

Max effort/breathing/pulse: _____

Core: _____

Stretching: _____

Successes: _____

Other: _____

Time/Distance/Totals, if any: _____

5

Date, day, time, location: _____

Feeling of energy/health before: _____during:_____ after: _____

Challenges: _____

Max effort/breathing/pulse: _____

Core: _____

Stretching: _____

Successes: _____

Other: _____

Time/Distance/Totals, if any: _____

6

Date, day, time, location: _____

Feeling of energy/health before: _____during:_____ after: _____

Challenges: _____

Max effort/breathing/pulse: _____

Core: _____

Stretching: _____

Successes: _____

Other: _____

Time/Distance/Totals, if any: _____

7

Date, day, time, location: _____

Feeling of energy/health before: _____during:_____ after: _____

Challenges: _____

Max effort/breathing/pulse: _____

Core: _____

Stretching: _____

Successes: _____

Other: _____

Time/Distance/Totals, if any: _____

8

Date, day, time, location: _____

Feeling of energy/health before: _____*during:*_____ *after:* _____

Challenges: _____

Max effort/breathing/pulse: _____

Core: _____

Stretching: _____

Successes: _____

Other: _____

Time/Distance/Totals, if any: _____

9

Date, day, time, location: _____

Feeling of energy/health before: _____*during:*_____ *after:* _____

Challenges: _____

Max effort/breathing/pulse: _____

Core: _____

Stretching: _____

Successes: _____

Other: _____

Time/Distance/Totals, if any: _____

10

Date, day, time, location: _____

Feeling of energy/health before: _____*during:*_____ *after:* _____

Challenges: _____

Max effort/breathing/pulse: _____

Core: _____

Stretching: _____

Successes: _____

Other: _____

Time/Distance/Totals, if any: _____

11

Date, day, time, location: _____

Feeling of energy/health before: _____*during:*_____ *after:* _____

Challenges: _____

Max effort/breathing/pulse: _____

Core: _____

Stretching: _____

Successes: _____

Other: _____

Time/Distance/Totals, if any: _____

12

Date, day, time, location: _____

Feeling of energy/health before: _____ *during:* _____ *after:* _____

Challenges: _____

Max effort/breathing/pulse: _____

Core: _____

Stretching: _____

Successes: _____

Other: _____

Time/Distance/Totals, if any: _____

13

Date, day, time, location: _____

Feeling of energy/health before: _____ *during:* _____ *after:* _____

Challenges: _____

Max effort/breathing/pulse: _____

Core: _____

Stretching: _____

Successes: _____

Other: _____

Time/Distance/Totals, if any: _____

14

Date, day, time, location: _____

Feeling of energy/health before: _____ *during:* _____ *after:* _____

Challenges: _____

Max effort/breathing/pulse: _____

Core: _____

Stretching: _____

Successes: _____

Other: _____

Time/Distance/Totals, if any: _____

15
Date, day, time, location: _____
Feeling of energy/health before: _____ *during:* _____ *after:* _____
Challenges: _____
Max effort/breathing/pulse: _____
Core: _____
Stretching: _____
Successes: _____
Other: _____
Time/Distance/Totals, if any: _____

16
Date, day, time, location: _____
Feeling of energy/health before: _____ *during:* _____ *after:* _____
Challenges: _____
Max effort/breathing/pulse: _____
Core: _____
Stretching: _____
Successes: _____
Other: _____
Time/Distance/Totals, if any: _____

17
Date, day, time, location: _____
Feeling of energy/health before: _____ *during:* _____ *after:* _____
Challenges: _____
Max effort/breathing/pulse: _____
Core: _____
Stretching: _____
Successes: _____
Other: _____
Time/Distance/Totals, if any: _____

18
Date, day, time, location: _____
Feeling of energy/health before: _____ *during:* _____ *after:* _____
Challenges: _____
Max effort/breathing/pulse: _____
Core: _____

Stretching: _____

Successes: _____

Other: _____

Time/Distance/Totals, if any: _____

19

Date, day, time, location: _____

Feeling of energy/health before: _____*during:*_____ *after:* _____

Challenges: _____

Max effort/breathing/pulse: _____

Core: _____

Stretching: _____

Successes: _____

Other: _____

Time/Distance/Totals, if any: _____

20

Date, day, time, location: _____

Feeling of energy/health before: _____*during:*_____ *after:* _____

Challenges: _____

Max effort/breathing/pulse: _____

Core: _____

Stretching: _____

Successes: _____

Other: _____

Time/Distance/Totals, if any: _____

21

Date, day, time, location: _____

Feeling of energy/health before: _____*during:*_____ *after:* _____

Challenges: _____

Max effort/breathing/pulse: _____

Core: _____

Stretching: _____

Successes: _____

Other: _____

Time/Distance/Totals, if any: _____

What shall I do today . . . heute . . . hoy . . . aujourd'hui . . . oggi . . . idag . . . tanaan . . . avui . . .

22
Date, day, time, location: _____
Feeling of energy/health before: _____during:_____ after: _____
Challenges: _____
Max effort/breathing/pulse: _____
Core: _____
Stretching: _____
Successes: _____
Other: _____
Time/Distance/Totals, if any: _____

23
Date, day, time, location: _____
Feeling of energy/health before: _____during:_____ after: _____
Challenges: _____
Max effort/breathing/pulse: _____
Core: _____
Stretching: _____
Successes: _____
Other: _____
Time/Distance/Totals, if any: _____

24
Date, day, time, location: _____
Feeling of energy/health before: _____during:_____ after: _____
Challenges: _____
Max effort/breathing/pulse: _____
Core: _____
Stretching: _____
Successes: _____
Other: _____
Time/Distance/Totals, if any: _____

25
Date, day, time, location: _____
Feeling of energy/health before: _____during:_____ after: _____
Challenges: _____
Max effort/breathing/pulse: _____
Core: _____

Stretching: _____

Successes: _____

Other: _____

Time/Distance/Totals, if any: _____

26

Date, day, time, location: _____

Feeling of energy/health before: _____during:_____ after: _____

Challenges: _____

Max effort/breathing/pulse: _____

Core: _____

Stretching: _____

Successes: _____

Other: _____

Time/Distance/Totals, if any: _____

27

Date, day, time, location: _____

Feeling of energy/health before: _____during:_____ after: _____

Challenges: _____

Max effort/breathing/pulse: _____

Core: _____

Stretching: _____

Successes: _____

Other: _____

Time/Distance/Totals, if any: _____

28

Date, day, time, location: _____

Feeling of energy/health before: _____during:_____ after: _____

Challenges: _____

Max effort/breathing/pulse: _____

Core: _____

Stretching: _____

Successes: _____

Other: _____

Time/Distance/Totals, if any: _____

29

Date, day, time, location: _____

Feeling of energy/health before: _____*during:*_____ *after:* _____

Challenges: _____

Max effort/breathing/pulse: _____

Core: _____

Stretching: _____

Successes: _____

Other: _____

Time/Distance/Totals, if any: _____

30

Date, day, time, location: _____

Feeling of energy/health before: _____*during:*_____ *after:* _____

Challenges: _____

Max effort/breathing/pulse: _____

Core: _____

Stretching: _____

Successes: _____

Other: _____

Time/Distance/Totals, if any: _____

31

Date, day, time, location: _____

Feeling of energy/health before: _____*during:*_____ *after:* _____

Challenges: _____

Max effort/breathing/pulse: _____

Core: _____

Stretching: _____

Successes: _____

Other: _____

Time/Distance/Totals, if any: _____

Extra Workouts 1

Date, day, time, location: _____

Feeling of energy/health before: _____during:_____ after: _____

Challenges: _____

Max effort/breathing/pulse: _____

Core: _____

Stretching: _____

Successes: _____

Other: _____

Time/Distance/Totals, if any: _____

Extra 2

Date, day, time, location: _____

Feeling of energy/health before: _____during:_____ after: _____

Challenges: _____ _____

Max effort/breathing/pulse: _____

Core: _____

Stretching: _____

Successes: _____

Other: _____

Time/Distance/Totals, if any: _____

Extra 3

Date, day, time, location: _____

Feeling of energy/health before: _____during:_____ after: _____

Challenges: _____

Max effort/breathing/pulse: _____

Core: _____

Stretching: _____

Successes: _____

Other: _____

Time/Distance/Totals, if any: _____

Extra 4

Date, day, time, location: _____

Feeling of energy/health before: _____during:_____ after: _____

Challenges: _____

Max effort/breathing/pulse: _____

Core: _____

What shall I do today . . . heute . . . hoy . . . aujourd'hui . . . oggi . . . idag . . . tanaan . . . avui . . .

Stretching: _____

Successes: _____

Other: _____

Time/Distance/Totals, if any: _____

Extra 5

Date, day, time, location: _____

Feeling of energy/health before: _____ *during:* _____ *after:* _____

Challenges: _____

Max effort/breathing/pulse: _____

Core: _____

Stretching: _____

Successes: _____

Other: _____

Time/Distance/Totals, if any: _____

End of Month Scoring

Method One: Basic (Number of days I exercised this month):_____
    Ultimate Goal: Every Day
    My Goal for This Month Was: _____
    My Goal for Next Month Is: _____
Method Two: Subtraction (Days I Rowed Minus Days Not):_____
    Initial Goal: Exceed Zero (row at least half the days)
    Ultimate Goal: Same as days in the month.
    My Goal for This Month Was: _____
    My Goal for Next Month Is: _____
Method Three: Division (Percentage = Days Rowed Divided by Total Days): _____
    Ultimate Goal: 100%
    My Goal for This Month Was:_____
    My Goal for Next Month Is: _____

Other Scores and Data for Month (Goals set and met; Times rowed; Distances rowed; Other):

_____

_____

_____

_____

_____

_____

_____

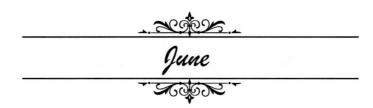

June

"To preserve health, we must do our exercises. Leisure hurts."
  Cristobal Mendez (Book of Bodily Exercise), Kolata, at 32

"Fat people who want to reduce should take their exercise on an empty stomach and sit down to their food out of breath . . . Thin people who want to get fat should do exactly the opposite and never take exercise on an empty stomach."
  Hippocrates

"The pure and simple reason why we exercise year after year is that it makes you feel good."
  Dr. Kenneth Cooper, Kolata, at 70

"Haskell [co-originator of the 220 minus your age maximum heart rate calculation] is a bit taken aback by the way the heart-rate formula has come to be viewed almost as a physical law. . . . When he and Fox proposed the formula . . . they never claimed to be providing a way to give a precise maximum heart rate for a given individual."
  Gina Kolata, at 89

Dr. Kenneth Cooper "decided he would apply the principles of scientific inquiry to decide how much exercise people really need to be healthy. . . . His questions were simple: Is walking one mile the same as running it? . . . No one really had a good answer."
  Gina Kolata, at 27

"Many people believe that exercise causes arthritis by placing stress on the joints. But in fact, moderate regular exercise often relieves arthritis pain and disability . . . ."
  Successful Aging, at 154

June – Stretching

Stretch every day.

The best time to stretch is shortly after exercise while your muscles are still warm. Many boathouses (and some gyms) do not have convenient areas set aside for stretching. Consider taking a yoga mat to stretch on. If you row at home, have a place to stretch as soon as you finish your row. If rowing elsewhere in a place you cannot stretch, try to get home quickly and stretch before showering. If that fails, consider doing some stretches before bed.

The motion of exercise involves alternately stretching out and then contracting the muscles that are powering the body. Complementary muscle groups move the body in one direction and then back, alternately stretching and contracting as the opposing muscles work together by working against them. Picture the arms during a slow push-up or pull-up or curl, for example.

One substantial challenge for a novice rower, and for anyone using muscles that have usually been dormant, is that muscles that contract when we use them tend to want to stay contracted; they may not readily loosen completely to allow the opposing muscles to work. That results in tightness that impairs your technique while rowing and can leave your muscles tighter and more sore after you exercise. You may feel warmed and relaxed when you finish rowing, but if you stop to stretch you will find that the muscles you were using are tightening. Happily, they can relax if given the opportunity. That is what stretching is all about – letting the muscles that just worked stretch out into a longer, relaxed position.

As for the stretching part of each motion during exercise, enjoy the way over time the muscles become more able to relax between contractions. The exercise itself, combined with after-exercise stretching, will give you a longer range of comfortable motion over time.

When you begin to stretch after exercise, focus on stretching the muscles you use. Since rowing is a full-body workout, this means there are many muscles you can stretch. Start with the big ones in the legs. Some rowers stretch some of the muscles they use but not all main muscle groups. We all tend to have a blind side in that way – doing what we are used to doing rather than what we need to work on the most. Think about what you are stretching. Try something different. Look for tight muscles and sore muscles and work on those, starting with the larger muscle groups – the hamstrings, the quads, and more.

Stretch to your comfort limit but not beyond. Stretching should be a challenge but should not hurt. And stretching takes time; your goal is to create comfortable resistance to tightening so that the muscles will relax and lengthen. Holding a position longer will do more good than stretching 'harder.' And you will find that as you hold a position longer, it will increase your ability to do a second stretch and reach farther with comfort after relaxing momentarily.

There are many places to find stretching exercises or routines. Take a yoga class (yoga postures rather than 'yoga-cize'), learn from the rowers at your club, look online, learn at sculling camp, learn from your rowing coach, check out books on the subject.

Ron had a well-developed routine of favorite stretches that he used and that he had taught to rowers he had coached. He had even been asked by parents of his junior rowers to offer a class for the parents and had found many were interested. In his own routine, he stretched religiously and kept it up right through races. He knew that it became even more important for him to stretch every day as he ratcheted up the intensity of his workouts.

Mel did not like to stretch. She did not like to sit or lie on the floor. And she was convinced that her very tight muscles were simply her nature. They had always felt this way and it seemed normal to her. She began to do a couple of stretches after she rowed. She found it frustrating. She did not feel her hamstrings lengthening out and felt it did nothing for her.

Andie used to feel the way Mel did and encouraged Mel to keep at it. Andie had found that it was only after she began to exercise more vigorously and got heated up more and even broke a sweat that she felt a difference when she stretched at the end of a workout. She still was not sure which muscles she ought to stretch or whether she was doing enough stretching, but she had begun to become familiar with the feeling that her muscles were becoming tighter as a result of her workouts. And she found that stretching felt relaxing and helped with that tightness and soreness.

1

Date, day, time, location: _____

Feeling of energy/health before: _____ *during:* _____ *after:* _____

Challenges: _____

Max effort/breathing/pulse: _____

Core: _____

Stretching: _____

Successes: _____

Other: _____

Time/Distance/Totals, if any: _____

2

Date, day, time, location: _____

Feeling of energy/health before: _____ *during:* _____ *after:* _____

Challenges: _____

Max effort/breathing/pulse: _____

Core: _____

Stretching: _____

Successes: _____

Other: _____

Time/Distance/Totals, if any: _____

3

Date, day, time, location: _____

Feeling of energy/health before: _____ *during:* _____ *after:* _____

Challenges: _____

Max effort/breathing/pulse: _____

Core: _____

Stretching: _____

Successes: _____

Other: _____

Time/Distance/Totals, if any: _____

4

Date, day, time, location: _____

Feeling of energy/health before: _____ *during:* _____ *after:* _____

Challenges: _____

Max effort/breathing/pulse: _____

Core: _____

What shall I do today . . . heute . . . hoy . . . aujourd'hui . . . oggi . . . idag . . . tanaan . . . avui . . .

Stretching: _____

Successes: _____

Other: _____

Time/Distance/Totals, if any: _____

5

Date, day, time, location: _____

Feeling of energy/health before: _____ *during:* _____ *after:* _____

Challenges: _____

Max effort/breathing/pulse: _____

Core: _____

Stretching: _____

Successes: _____

Other: _____

Time/Distance/Totals, if any: _____

6

Date, day, time, location: _____

Feeling of energy/health before: _____ *during:* _____ *after:* _____

Challenges: _____

Max effort/breathing/pulse: _____

Core: _____

Stretching: _____

Successes: _____

Other: _____

Time/Distance/Totals, if any: _____

7

Date, day, time, location: _____

Feeling of energy/health before: _____ *during:* _____ *after:* _____

Challenges: _____

Max effort/breathing/pulse: _____

Core: _____

Stretching: _____

Successes: _____

Other: _____

Time/Distance/Totals, if any: _____

8

Date, day, time, location: _____

Feeling of energy/health before: _____during:_____ after: _____

Challenges: _____

Max effort/breathing/pulse: _____

Core: _____

Stretching: _____

Successes: _____

Other: _____

Time/Distance/Totals, if any: _____

9

Date, day, time, location: _____

Feeling of energy/health before: _____during:_____ after: _____

Challenges: _____

Max effort/breathing/pulse: _____

Core: _____

Stretching: _____

Successes: _____

Other: _____

Time/Distance/Totals, if any: _____

10

Date, day, time, location: _____

Feeling of energy/health before: _____during:_____ after: _____

Challenges: _____

Max effort/breathing/pulse: _____

Core: _____

Stretching: _____

Successes: _____

Other: _____

Time/Distance/Totals, if any: _____

11

Date, day, time, location: _____

Feeling of energy/health before: _____during:_____ after: _____

Challenges: _____

Max effort/breathing/pulse: _____

Core: _____

What shall I do today . . . heute . . . hoy . . . aujourd'hui . . . oggi . . . idag . . . tanaan . . . avui . . .

Stretching: _____

Successes: _____

Other: _____

Time/Distance/Totals, if any: _____

12

Date, day, time, location: _____

Feeling of energy/health before: _____ *during:* _____ *after:* _____

Challenges: _____

Max effort/breathing/pulse: _____

Core: _____

Stretching: _____

Successes: _____

Other: _____

Time/Distance/Totals, if any: _____

13

Date, day, time, location: _____

Feeling of energy/health before: _____ *during:* _____ *after:* _____

Challenges: _____

Max effort/breathing/pulse: _____

Core: _____

Stretching: _____

Successes: _____

Other: _____

Time/Distance/Totals, if any: _____

14

Date, day, time, location: _____

Feeling of energy/health before: _____ *during:* _____ *after:* _____

Challenges: _____

Max effort/breathing/pulse: _____

Core: _____

Stretching: _____

Successes: _____

Other: _____

Time/Distance/Totals, if any: _____

15

Date, day, time, location: _____

Feeling of energy/health before: _____ *during:* _____ *after:* _____

Challenges: _____

Max effort/breathing/pulse: _____

Core: _____

Stretching: _____

Successes: _____

Other: _____

Time/Distance/Totals, if any: _____

16

Date, day, time, location: _____

Feeling of energy/health before: _____ *during:* _____ *after:* _____

Challenges: _____

Max effort/breathing/pulse: _____

Core: _____

Stretching: _____

Successes: _____

Other: _____

Time/Distance/Totals, if any: _____

17

Date, day, time, location: _____

Feeling of energy/health before: _____ *during:* _____ *after:* _____

Challenges: _____

Max effort/breathing/pulse: _____

Core: _____

Stretching: _____

Successes: _____

Other: _____

Time/Distance/Totals, if any: _____

18

Date, day, time, location: _____

Feeling of energy/health before: _____ *during:* _____ *after:* _____

Challenges: _____

Max effort/breathing/pulse: _____

Core: _____

What shall I do today . . . heute . . . hoy . . . aujourd'hui . . . oggi . . . idag . . . tanaan . . . avui . . .

Stretching: _____

Successes: _____

Other: _____

Time/Distance/Totals, if any: _____

19

Date, day, time, location: _____

Feeling of energy/health before: _____ *during:* _____ *after:* _____

Challenges: _____

Max effort/breathing/pulse: _____

Core: _____

Stretching: _____

Successes: _____

Other: _____

Time/Distance/Totals, if any: _____

20

Date, day, time, location: _____

Feeling of energy/health before: _____ *during:* _____ *after:* _____

Challenges: _____

Max effort/breathing/pulse: _____

Core: _____

Stretching: _____

Successes: _____

Other: _____

Time/Distance/Totals, if any: _____

21

Date, day, time, location: _____

Feeling of energy/health before: _____ *during:* _____ *after:* _____

Challenges: _____

Max effort/breathing/pulse: _____

Core: _____

Stretching: _____

Successes: _____

Other: _____

Time/Distance/Totals, if any: _____

22

Date, day, time, location: _____
Feeling of energy/health before: _____ *during:* _____ *after:* _____
Challenges: _____ _ _____
Max effort/breathing/pulse: _____
Core: _____
Stretching: _____
Successes: _____
Other: _____
Time/Distance/Totals, if any: _____

23

Date, day, time, location: _____
Feeling of energy/health before: _____ *during:* _____ *after:* _____
Challenges: _____
Max effort/breathing/pulse: _____
Core: _____
Stretching: _____
Successes: _____
Other: _____
Time/Distance/Totals, if any: _____

24

Date, day, time, location: _____
Feeling of energy/health before: _____ *during:* _____ *after:* _____
Challenges: _____
Max effort/breathing/pulse: _____
Core: _____
Stretching: _____
Successes: _____
Other: _____
Time/Distance/Totals, if any: _____

25

Date, day, time, location: _____
Feeling of energy/health before: _____ *during:* _____ *after:* _____
Challenges: _____
Max effort/breathing/pulse: _____
Core: _____

Stretching: _____

Successes: _____

Other: _____

Time/Distance/Totals, if any: _____

26

Date, day, time, location: _____

Feeling of energy/health before: _____*during:*_____ *after:* _____

Challenges: _____

Max effort/breathing/pulse: _____

Core: _____

Stretching: _____

Successes: _____

Other: _____

Time/Distance/Totals, if any: _____

27

Date, day, time, location: _____

Feeling of energy/health before: _____*during:*_____ *after:* _____

Challenges: _____

Max effort/breathing/pulse: _____

Core: _____

Stretching: _____

Successes: _____

Other: _____

Time/Distance/Totals, if any: _____

28

Date, day, time, location: _____

Feeling of energy/health before: _____*during:*_____ *after:* _____

Challenges: _____

Max effort/breathing/pulse: _____

Core: _____

Stretching: _____

Successes: _____

Other: _____

Time/Distance/Totals, if any: _____

29

Date, day, time, location: _____

Feeling of energy/health before: _____ *during:* _____ *after:* _____

Challenges: _____

Max effort/breathing/pulse: _____

Core: _____

Stretching: _____

Successes: _____

Other: _____

Time/Distance/Totals, if any: _____

30

Date, day, time, location: _____

Feeling of energy/health before: _____ *during:* _____ *after:* _____

Challenges: _____

Max effort/breathing/pulse: _____

Core: _____

Stretching: _____

Successes: _____

Other: _____

Time/Distance/Totals, if any: _____

31

Date, day, time, location: _____

Feeling of energy/health before: _____ *during:* _____ *after:* _____

Challenges: _____

Max effort/breathing/pulse: _____

Core: _____

Stretching: _____

Successes: _____

Other: _____

Time/Distance/Totals, if any: _____

What shall I do today . . . heute . . . hoy . . . aujourd'hui . . . oggi . . . idag . . . tanaan . . . avui . . .

Extra Workouts 1
Date, day, time, location: _____
Feeling of energy/health before: _____ during: _____ after: _____
Challenges: _____
Max effort/breathing/pulse: _____
Core: _____
Stretching: _____
Successes: _____
Other: _____
Time/Distance/Totals, if any: _____

Extra 2
Date, day, time, location: _____
Feeling of energy/health before: _____ during: _____ after: _____
Challenges: _____
Max effort/breathing/pulse: _____
Core: _____
Stretching: _____
Successes: _____
Other: _____
Time/Distance/Totals, if any: _____

Extra 3
Date, day, time, location: _____
Feeling of energy/health before: _____ during: _____ after: _____
Challenges: _____
Max effort/breathing/pulse: _____
Core: _____
Stretching: _____
Successes: _____
Other: _____
Time/Distance/Totals, if any: _____

Extra 4
Date, day, time, location: _____
Feeling of energy/health before: _____ during: _____ after: _____
Challenges: _____
Max effort/breathing/pulse: _____
Core: _____

Stretching: _____

Successes: _____

Other: _____

Time/Distance/Totals, if any: _____

Extra 5

Date, day, time, location: _____

Feeling of energy/health before: _____ during: _____ after: _____

Challenges: _____ . _____

Max effort/breathing/pulse: _____

Core: _____

Stretching: _____

Successes: _____

Other: _____

Time/Distance/Totals, if any: _____

End of Month Scoring

Method One: Basic (Number of days I exercised this month):_____
    Ultimate Goal: Every Day
    My Goal for This Month Was: _____
    My Goal for Next Month Is: _____
Method Two: Subtraction (Days I Rowed Minus Days Not):_____
    Initial Goal: Exceed Zero (row at least half the days)
    Ultimate Goal: Same as days in the month.
    My Goal for This Month Was: _____
    My Goal for Next Month Is: _____
Method Three: Division (Percentage = Days Rowed Divided by Total Days): _____
    Ultimate Goal: 100%
    My Goal for This Month Was:_____
    My Goal for Next Month Is: _____

Other Scores and Data for Month (Goals set and met; Times rowed; Distances rowed; Other):

_____

_____

_____

_____

_____

_____

_____

Season Recap and Change

Scoring

You have calculated your score at the end of each month. Take a season-long look at your progress. Where have you improved during the three months of this season? Compare season to season as the year progresses. Most importantly, once you calculate your score, consider whether it correlates with how you feel.

_____

_____

_____

_____

Goals Accomplished

Look back on your goals for the past season. Did you set goals based on how many days you rowed? Did you set goals to row longer or harder each day? If you are succeeding with both of those challenges, how are you doing at including core work and stretching each day? (Are you keeping track of that?) Do you also set goals for distances rowed or pace? Have you planned to take a rowing class or attend a rowing event? For these and other goals you may have set three months ago, look back and record here how you did.

_____

_____

_____

_____

_____

_____

Goals Looking Ahead

Once you have looked back, plan ahead. Set some goals. Make them realistic based on your past experience, events coming up and your other plans for the coming three months.

_____

_____

_____

_____

_____

Changes for Variety

Do you cross-train for variety? How can you modify that in the coming season? Plan a vacation based on doing something active you would enjoy. Add an aerobics or spinning or pilates class or some weight lifting or yoga or something else you may not normally do.

_____

_____

_____

_____

_____

July

"Patients should have rest, food, fresh air, and exercise – the quadrangle of health."
   Sir William Osler, MD (1849-1919)

"The will to win means nothing without the will to prepare."
   Juma Ikangaa (Tanzanian marathoner)

"[T]he pace of aging varies with heredity, environment, and the level of physical activity."
   Encyclopedia, at 583

"Many of the elderly are paying a high price (poor health and premature mortality) because they were not physically active as their bodies aged. Exercise can help slow the decline in muscle strength and flexibility and may even improve the functional status of many organ systems."
   Encyclopedia, at 584

"A sedentary lifestyle, in conjunction with poor health habits, may contribute to the deterioration commonly associated with aging. By contrast, the benefits of regular exercise include improved self-esteem, higher ratio of lean muscle tissue to fat and bone mineral mass, a stronger cardiovascular system, improved reaction time and balance, stronger muscles and tendons, and possibly improvements in memory, judgment, control of urination, absorption and metabolization of drugs, and gastrointestinal function.
   Encyclopedia, at 596-97

July – Race or Volunteer at Club Regattas

For many rowing clubs, summer and fall are club racing seasons (whereas the spring is racing season for junior crews and college teams). Summer regattas involve shorter, sprint racing (usually 1,000 to 2,000 meters long), with opportunities to participate for rowers of all ages (and experience – there often are 'novice' events). Fall racing is usually 'head' racing, with a standard distance of three miles (or five kilometers) if the venue allows for it. While summer racing involves rowers starting next to one another and racing to the finish line on the starter's command, head racing has each rower begin alone and race against the clock. Since you start only a few seconds apart in a head race, it is common for some racers to pass others. But the fall racing may feel more like you are pitting your skills against the river instead of primarily the other rowers because you are not side by side at the starting line. Like summer racing, many fall head race regattas include a novice event. And masters (older racers) are allowed to race (or at least be scored) according to their age group. Consider racing if you want a challenge. You do not have to seek to win or place for racing to be a beneficial goal. Merely planning to participate will have an effect on your training.

These regattas are great opportunities to get to know rowing club members and to help the club serve the community. Since regattas are staffed mostly (if not entirely) by volunteers, there is always a need for more help. Some jobs can be done by anyone, from setting up tables or tents to helping with cleanup at the end. Many tasks can be done with minimal training, including helping with registration, driving a launch and helping with other organizational tasks. And the jobs that require more background or training, like serving as a starter or referee or finish line judge, are often jobs that clubs will provide training for.

Getting to know other rowers is a great way to supplement your individual training. Most rowers are supportive people and want to encourage novice rowers. Since club officials love to have more help, they usually will respond to your interest with a desire to share what they know about rowing as well as to involve you in the regatta planning and hosting. Be warned that you may experience what may seem like a standoffish or superior attitude from some competitive rowers. To many, 'true rowing' is kind of like religion and some may expect you to embrace competitive rowing unreservedly or hold you in lower esteem if you do not. They might say that rowing is only true rowing if you are in fantastic condition and pushing yourself to your limits when competing. But the simple truth is that the rowing motion and the benefits of rowing are accessible to all, whether or not you are planning to compete, whether or not you are in superb physical condition, and whether or not you are highly skilled at rowing. So on the rare occasion when you meet one of these elitists, shrug it off. And keep in mind that often the toughest competitors are not elitist at all, but rather are among the many who welcome beginners of all backgrounds.

With the exception of the larger regattas that may go on for two or more days, most summer and fall regattas are a one day affair. The planning may go on for months, but you as a volunteer will not need to be that involved unless you join the planning committee. Volunteering will likely take only a few hours on one day – before the race day if you are helping to set up the course, for example, but usually on the day of the regatta.

And if, once you become a volunteer, you decide to race, the others in the club will usually be able to help you work with your volunteer schedule so that volunteering does not get in the way of racing.

Ron has been involved in the planning and hosting of many regattas, as well as racing at many venues for more than twenty years. He has passed on many of the organizational duties to others, but still is willing to volunteer and to work with other volunteers.

Mel does not feel ready to race, even in a novice event. But she has signed up to help with the main tent at the local July regatta. There she will help with race information and support other volunteers as they answer questions by coaches, competitors and spectators in order to help regatta officials run a smooth regatta.

Andie took the spring learn-to-row class on the river in May after taking intermediate indoor rowing in February. She enjoyed rowing with the 30 or so other novices and joined an eight who wanted to enter the novice event at the July regatta. So she is planning to race and to limit her volunteering to helping with cleanup.

What shall I do today . . . heute . . . hoy . . . aujourd'hui . . . oggi . . . idag . . . tanaan . . . avui . . .

1

Date, day, time, location: _____

Feeling of energy/health before: _____ during: _____ after: _____

Challenges: _____

Max effort/breathing/pulse: _____

Core: _____

Stretching: _____

Successes: _____

Other: _____

Time/Distance/Totals, if any: _____

2

Date, day, time, location: _____

Feeling of energy/health before: _____ during: _____ after: _____

Challenges: _____

Max effort/breathing/pulse: _____

Core: _____

Stretching: _____

Successes: _____

Other: _____

Time/Distance/Totals, if any: _____

3

Date, day, time, location: _____

Feeling of energy/health before: _____ during: _____ after: _____

Challenges: _____

Max effort/breathing/pulse: _____

Core: _____

Stretching: _____

Successes: _____

Other: _____

Time/Distance/Totals, if any: _____

4

Date, day, time, location: _____

Feeling of energy/health before: _____ during: _____ after: _____

Challenges: _____

Max effort/breathing/pulse: _____

Core: _____

Stretching: _____

Successes: _____

Other: _____

Time/Distance/Totals, if any: _____

5

Date, day, time, location: _____

Feeling of energy/health before: _____during:_____ after: _____

Challenges: _____

Max effort/breathing/pulse: _____

Core: _____

Stretching: _____

Successes: _____

Other: _____

Time/Distance/Totals, if any: _____

6

Date, day, time, location: _____

Feeling of energy/health before: _____during:_____ after: _____

Challenges: _____

Max effort/breathing/pulse: _____

Core: _____

Stretching: _____

Successes: _____

Other: _____

Time/Distance/Totals, if any: _____

7

Date, day, time, location: _____

Feeling of energy/health before: _____during:_____ after: _____

Challenges: _____

Max effort/breathing/pulse: _____

Core: _____

Stretching: _____

Successes: _____

Other: _____

Time/Distance/Totals, if any: _____

8

Date, day, time, location: _____

Feeling of energy/health before: _____*during:*_____ *after:* _____

Challenges: _____

Max effort/breathing/pulse: _____

Core: _____

Stretching: _____

Successes: _____

Other: _____

Time/Distance/Totals, if any: _____

9

Date, day, time, location: _____

Feeling of energy/health before: _____*during:*_____ *after:* _____

Challenges: _____

Max effort/breathing/pulse: _____

Core: _____

Stretching: _____

Successes: _____

Other: _____

Time/Distance/Totals, if any: _____

10

Date, day, time, location: _____

Feeling of energy/health before: _____*during:*_____ *after:* _____

Challenges: _____

Max effort/breathing/pulse: _____

Core: _____

Stretching: _____

Successes: _____

Other: _____

Time/Distance/Totals, if any: _____

11

Date, day, time, location: _____

Feeling of energy/health before: _____*during:*_____ *after:* _____

Challenges: _____

Max effort/breathing/pulse: _____

Core: _____

Stretching: _____

Successes: _____

Other: _____

Time/Distance/Totals, if any: _____

12

Date, day, time, location: _____

Feeling of energy/health before: _____*during:*_____ *after:* _____

Challenges: _____

Max effort/breathing/pulse: _____

Core: _____

Stretching: _____

Successes: _____

Other: _____

Time/Distance/Totals, if any: _____

13

Date, day, time, location: _____

Feeling of energy/health before: _____*during:*_____ *after:* _____

Challenges: _____

Max effort/breathing/pulse: _____

Core: _____

Stretching: _____

Successes: _____

Other: _____

Time/Distance/Totals, if any: _____

14

Date, day, time, location: _____

Feeling of energy/health before: _____*during:*_____ *after:* _____

Challenges: _____

Max effort/breathing/pulse: _____

Core: _____

Stretching: _____

Successes: _____

Other: _____

Time/Distance/Totals, if any: _____

15

Date, day, time, location: _____

Feeling of energy/health before: _____*during:*_____ *after:* _____

Challenges: _____

Max effort/breathing/pulse: _____

Core: _____

Stretching: _____

Successes: _____

Other: _____

Time/Distance/Totals, if any: _____

16

Date, day, time, location: _____

Feeling of energy/health before: _____*during:*_____ *after:* _____

Challenges: _____

Max effort/breathing/pulse: _____

Core: _____

Stretching: _____

Successes: _____

Other: _____

Time/Distance/Totals, if any: _____

17

Date, day, time, location: _____

Feeling of energy/health before: _____*during:*_____ *after:* _____

Challenges: _____

Max effort/breathing/pulse: _____

Core: _____

Stretching: _____

Successes: _____

Other: _____

Time/Distance/Totals, if any: _____

18

Date, day, time, location: _____

Feeling of energy/health before: _____*during:*_____ *after:* _____

Challenges: _____

Max effort/breathing/pulse: _____

Core: _____

Stretching: _____ _____

Successes: _____

Other: _____

Time/Distance/Totals, if any: _____

19

Date, day, time, location: _____

Feeling of energy/health before: _____during:_____ after: _____

Challenges: _____

Max effort/breathing/pulse: _____

Core: _____

Stretching: _____

Successes: _____

Other: _____

Time/Distance/Totals, if any: _____

20

Date, day, time, location: _____

Feeling of energy/health before: _____during:_____ after: _____

Challenges: _____

Max effort/breathing/pulse: _____

Core: _____

Stretching: _____

Successes: _____

Other: _____

Time/Distance/Totals, if any: _____

21

Date, day, time, location: _____

Feeling of energy/health before: _____during:_____ after: _____

Challenges: _____

Max effort/breathing/pulse: _____

Core: _____ _____

Stretching: _____ _____

Successes: _____ _____

Other: _____ _____

Time/Distance/Totals, if any: _____

What shall I do today . . . heute . . . hoy . . . aujourd'hui . . . oggi . . . idag . . . tanaan . . . avui . . .

22

Date, day, time, location: _____

Feeling of energy/health before: _____ *during:* _____ *after:* _____

Challenges: _____

Max effort/breathing/pulse: _____

Core: _____

Stretching: _____

Successes: _____

Other: _____

Time/Distance/Totals, if any: _____

23

Date, day, time, location: _____

Feeling of energy/health before: _____ *during:* _____ *after:* _____

Challenges: _____

Max effort/breathing/pulse: _____

Core: _____

Stretching: _____

Successes: _____

Other: _____

Time/Distance/Totals, if any: _____

24

Date, day, time, location: _____

Feeling of energy/health before: _____ *during:* _____ *after:* _____

Challenges: _____

Max effort/breathing/pulse: _____

Core: _____

Stretching: _____

Successes: _____

Other: _____

Time/Distance/Totals, if any: _____

25

Date, day, time, location: _____

Feeling of energy/health before: _____ *during:* _____ *after:* _____

Challenges: _____

Max effort/breathing/pulse: _____

Core: _____

Stretching: _____

Successes: _____

Other: _____

Time/Distance/Totals, if any: _____

26

Date, day, time, location: _____

Feeling of energy/health before: _____ during:_____ after: _____

Challenges: _____

Max effort/breathing/pulse: _____

Core: _____

Stretching: _____

Successes: _____

Other: _____

Time/Distance/Totals, if any: _____

27

Date, day, time, location: _____

Feeling of energy/health before: _____ during:_____ after: _____

Challenges: _____

Max effort/breathing/pulse: _____

Core: _____

Stretching: _____

Successes: _____

Other: _____

Time/Distance/Totals, if any: _____

28

Date, day, time, location: _____

Feeling of energy/health before: _____ during:_____ after: _____

Challenges: _____

Max effort/breathing/pulse: _____

Core: _____

Stretching: _____

Successes: _____

Other: _____

Time/Distance/Totals, if any: _____

29

Date, day, time, location: _____

Feeling of energy/health before: _____during:_____ after: _____

Challenges: _____

Max effort/breathing/pulse: _____

Core: _____

Stretching: _____

Successes: _____

Other: _____

Time/Distance/Totals, if any: _____

30

Date, day, time, location: _____

Feeling of energy/health before: _____during:_____ after: _____

Challenges: _____

Max effort/breathing/pulse: _____

Core: _____

Stretching: _____

Successes: _____

Other: _____

Time/Distance/Totals, if any: _____

31

Date, day, time, location: _____

Feeling of energy/health before: _____during:_____ after: _____

Challenges: _____

Max effort/breathing/pulse: _____

Core: _____

Stretching: _____

Successes: _____

Other: _____

Time/Distance/Totals, if any: _____

Extra Workouts 1

Date, day, time, location: _____

Feeling of energy/health before: _____during:_____ after: _____

Challenges: _____

Max effort/breathing/pulse: _____

Core: _____

Stretching: _____

Successes: _____

Other: _____

Time/Distance/Totals, if any: _____

Extra 2

Date, day, time, location: _____

Feeling of energy/health before: _____during:_____ after: _____

Challenges: _____

Max effort/breathing/pulse: _____

Core: _____

Stretching: _____

Successes: _____

Other: _____

Time/Distance/Totals, if any: _____

Extra 3

Date, day, time, location: _____

Feeling of energy/health before: _____during:_____ after: _____

Challenges: _____

Max effort/breathing/pulse: _____

Core: _____

Stretching: _____

Successes: _____

Other: _____

Time/Distance/Totals, if any: _____

Extra 4

Date, day, time, location: _____

Feeling of energy/health before: _____during:_____ after: _____

Challenges: _____

Max effort/breathing/pulse: _____

Core: _____

What shall I do today . . . heute . . . hoy . . . aujourd'hui . . . oggi . . . idag . . . tanaan . . . avui . . .

Stretching: _____

Successes: _____

Other: _____

Time/Distance/Totals, if any: _____

Extra 5

Date, day, time, location: _____

Feeling of energy/health before: _____ *during:* _____ *after:* _____

Challenges: _____

Max effort/breathing/pulse: _____

Core: _____

Stretching: _____

Successes: _____

Other: _____

Time/Distance/Totals, if any: _____

End of Month Scoring

Method One: Basic (Number of days I exercised this month):_____
    Ultimate Goal: Every Day
    My Goal for This Month Was: _____
    My Goal for Next Month Is: _____

Method Two: Subtraction (Days I Rowed Minus Days Not):_____
    Initial Goal: Exceed Zero (row at least half the days)
    Ultimate Goal: Same as days in the month.
    My Goal for This Month Was: _____
    My Goal for Next Month Is: _____

Method Three: Division (Percentage = Days Rowed Divided by Total Days): _____
    Ultimate Goal: 100%
    My Goal for This Month Was:_____
    My Goal for Next Month Is: _____

Other Scores and Data for Month (Goals set and met; Times rowed; Distances rowed; Other):

_____

_____

_____

_____

_____

_____

_____

August

"We do not stop exercising because we grow old; we grow old because we stop exercising."
  Dr. Kenneth Cooper

"Older people may have many concerns about exercising. . . . too old to start . . . too many aches and pains . . . fear injury . . . . However, these obstacles can be overcome. In fact, exercise can reduce them. It can make people feel younger and better."
  Merck, at 806

"While the benefits of regular exercise on lung function are numerous, the most significant result is increased efficiency of the lungs. Increasing lung efficiency and tidal volume [the volume of air breathed in per breath] through physical activity and exercise allows for a much more active lifestyle without undue respiratory stress."
  Encyclopedia, at 590

"For both excessive and insufficient exercise destroy one's strength, and both eating and drinking too much or too little destroy health, whereas the right quantity produces, increases and preserves it. . . . This much then, is clear: in all our conduct it is the mean that is to be commended."
  Aristotle (384-322 BC)

"[T]hose who sit at their work and are therefore called 'chair workers' . . . suffer from general ill-health and an excessive accumulation of unwholesome humors caused by their sedentary life."
  Bernardino Ramazzini (1713)

"To be aerobic, exercise must be continued for at least 20 minutes, according to many experts. Walking, running, biking, rowing, swimming, dancing, and skating are aerobic exercise. Aerobic exercise should be done 3 to 7 times a week."
  Merck, at 809

August – Rowing Tourism

Many of us masters rowers look for opportunities to row when we go on vacation. Some rowing clubs welcome visitors or 'tourists.' You may want to arrange to borrow equipment, sub in to a masters rowing group, or take your single with you and get out on the local river or lake where you vacation. Often a little advance planning is all it takes.

Have a vacation home? Then you may have a single already waiting for you there at the lake. You are lucky. You can roll out of bed and go out to the boat rack in your yard and go for a row. You may be back from your row sipping another cup of coffee before others in the house are even up.

Have you gone to sculling camp? If so, you have experienced the relaxation of rowing, eating and sleeping, as well as the enjoyment of sharing the experience with other rowers of all ages and levels of experience. Turn off the modern world and get away from it to row. (And, by the way, how can anyone worry about whether rowing every day is too much when you row three times a day at camp and *that* feels good?)

Or, perhaps you have toured Europe or other parts of the world for a rowing experience. There are tour companies working with rowing coaches who offer unusual experiences around the world for the vacationing rower.

But have you ever simply gone out of your way to find a lake or river you have never rowed on so you can experience it? The outdoor rowing experience is not just about driving the legs and handling the oar while balancing the boat, although that is enough to make it an experience that benefits from concentration. It is also about becoming more attuned to the weather and seeing a side of nature few others see. The vegetation and wildlife along rivers and lakes can be complex and ever-changing. Consider taking a rowing vacation with your single on the car and no boathouse stops scheduled. Where might you go to try new water, famous rivers, well-known lakes, normally un-rowed waters?

Some states like Minnesota and Michigan are riddled with many small lakes and streams, many rowable for at least part of their length and many with state-operated boat launch areas. While these boat launches are usually designed for and used primarily by fishermen backing their motor boats into the water, they can be great spots to wet launch your single. Or try the inland waterways in the south, protected lakes in the Rockies and Sierras, the great historic rivers like the Connecticut River, the Hudson River, the Ohio River, the upper Mississippi, and other major rivers and their tributaries. Much of the length of some of these rivers, like the massive Mississippi or the Amazon or even the lower Hudson, might not be safe or enjoyable to row in your racing single because of the size of open water and the effects of wind and weather together with current (and tides). But farther upriver, there may be miles of good, rowable water.

A different idea that may take more planning is rowing a series of city rivers. Many cities were originally located where they are in part because of the presence of navigable water. Rowing centers like Boston, Philadelphia, and Washington are easy choices with many boathouses that may (or may not) allow you to use their docks. Consider developing a plan to row the rivers in several other major cities, such as New York, London, Paris, Basel, Vienna, Budapest. Consider smaller cities and rural areas with rivers you can row on. Can you recommend rivers around the world to fellow rowers interested in rowing tourism?

And, of course, there are many great open water boats that can help you enjoy the larger rivers, the Great Lakes, and the oceans (and the bays, sounds and harbors along the ocean). Row Puget Sound, San Francisco Bay, and many other destinations. Just plan ahead, have the right equipment for the conditions, learn about local wind, weather, tide and water concerns. And bring backup, preferably a fellow rower and/or someone on shore who knows where you are at all times.

Ron participated in a marathon group row in Europe. It was a different form of training and an unusual experience. He has also participated in long road tours as an incentive to maintain a higher level of cross-training.

Mel visits her Grandparents on a lake up north each summer. She used to see one of the neighbors out rowing some early mornings as she drank her coffee, but never thought about doing it herself. Now she is going to ask if he still has his single and find out whether he would let her use it.

Andie and a friend who taught her to scull are going to tour New England next summer. They are looking into B&Bs near bodies of water and planning to take their boats on the car with them (assuming Andie gets her own single by then).

1

Date, day, time, location: _____

Feeling of energy/health before: _____*during:*_____ *after:* _____

Challenges: _____

Max effort/breathing/pulse: _____

Core: _____

Stretching: _____

Successes: _____

Other: _____

Time/Distance/Totals, if any: _____

2

Date, day, time, location: _____

Feeling of energy/health before: _____*during:*_____ *after:* _____

Challenges: _____

Max effort/breathing/pulse: _____

Core: _____

Stretching: _____

Successes: _____

Other: _____

Time/Distance/Totals, if any: _____

3

Date, day, time, location: _____

Feeling of energy/health before: _____*during:*_____ *after:* _____

Challenges: _____

Max effort/breathing/pulse: _____

Core: _____

Stretching: _____

Successes: _____

Other: _____

Time/Distance/Totals, if any: _____

4

Date, day, time, location: _____

Feeling of energy/health before: _____*during:*_____ *after:* _____

Challenges: _____

Max effort/breathing/pulse: _____

Core: _____

Stretching: _____

Successes: _____

Other: _____

Time/Distance/Totals, if any: _____

5

Date, day, time, location: _____

Feeling of energy/health before: _____ during: _____ after: _____

Challenges: _____

Max effort/breathing/pulse: _____

Core: _____

Stretching: _____

Successes: _____

Other: _____

Time/Distance/Totals, if any: _____

6

Date, day, time, location: _____

Feeling of energy/health before: _____ during: _____ after: _____

Challenges: _____

Max effort/breathing/pulse: _____

Core: _____

Stretching: _____

Successes: _____

Other: _____

Time/Distance/Totals, if any: _____

7

Date, day, time, location: _____

Feeling of energy/health before: _____ during: _____ after: _____

Challenges: _____

Max effort/breathing/pulse: _____

Core: _____

Stretching: _____

Successes: _____

Other: _____

Time/Distance/Totals, if any: _____

8

Date, day, time, location: _____

Feeling of energy/health before: _____ *during:* _____ *after:* _____

Challenges: _____

Max effort/breathing/pulse: _____

Core: _____

Stretching: _____

Successes: _____

Other: _____

Time/Distance/Totals, if any: _____

9

Date, day, time, location: _____

Feeling of energy/health before: _____ *during:* _____ *after:* _____

Challenges: _____

Max effort/breathing/pulse: _____

Core: _____

Stretching: _____

Successes: _____

Other: _____

Time/Distance/Totals, if any: _____

10

Date, day, time, location: _____

Feeling of energy/health before: _____ *during:* _____ *after:* _____

Challenges: _____

Max effort/breathing/pulse: _____

Core: _____

Stretching: _____

Successes: _____

Other: _____

Time/Distance/Totals, if any: _____

11

Date, day, time, location: _____

Feeling of energy/health before: _____ *during:* _____ *after:* _____

Challenges: _____

Max effort/breathing/pulse: _____

Core: _____

Stretching: _____

Successes: _____

Other: _____

Time/Distance/Totals, if any: _____

12

Date, day, time, location: _____

Feeling of energy/health before: _____ *during:* _____ *after:* _____

Challenges: _____

Max effort/breathing/pulse: _____

Core: _____

Stretching: _____

Successes: _____

Other: _____

Time/Distance/Totals, if any: _____

13

Date, day, time, location: _____

Feeling of energy/health before: _____ *during:* _____ *after:* _____

Challenges: _____

Max effort/breathing/pulse: _____

Core: _____

Stretching: _____

Successes: _____

Other: _____

Time/Distance/Totals, if any: _____

14

Date, day, time, location: _____

Feeling of energy/health before: _____ *during:* _____ *after:* _____

Challenges: _____

Max effort/breathing/pulse: _____

Core: _____

Stretching: _____

Successes: _____

Other: _____

Time/Distance/Totals, if any: _____

15

Date, day, time, location: _____
Feeling of energy/health before: _____during:_____ after: _____
Challenges: _____
Max effort/breathing/pulse: _____
Core: _____
Stretching: _____
Successes: _____
Other: _____
Time/Distance/Totals, if any: _____

16

Date, day, time, location: _____
Feeling of energy/health before: _____during:_____ after: _____
Challenges: _____
Max effort/breathing/pulse: _____
Core: _____
Stretching: _____
Successes: _____
Other: _____
Time/Distance/Totals, if any: _____

17

Date, day, time, location: _____
Feeling of energy/health before: _____during:_____ after: _____
Challenges: _____
Max effort/breathing/pulse: _____
Core: _____
Stretching: _____
Successes: _____
Other: _____
Time/Distance/Totals, if any: _____

18

Date, day, time, location: _____
Feeling of energy/health before: _____during:_____ after: _____
Challenges: _____
Max effort/breathing/pulse: _____
Core: _____

What shall I do today . . . heute . . . hoy . . . aujourd'hui . . . oggi . . . idag . . . tanaan . . . avui . . .

Stretching: _____

Successes: _____

Other: _____

Time/Distance/Totals, if any: _____

19

Date, day, time, location: _____

Feeling of energy/health before: _____during:_____ after: _____

Challenges: _____

Max effort/breathing/pulse: _____

Core: _____

Stretching: _____

Successes: _____

Other: _____

Time/Distance/Totals, if any: _____

20

Date, day, time, location: _____

Feeling of energy/health before: _____during:_____ after: _____

Challenges: _____

Max effort/breathing/pulse: _____

Core: _____

Stretching: _____

Successes: _____

Other: _____

Time/Distance/Totals, if any: _____

21

Date, day, time, location: _____

Feeling of energy/health before: _____during:_____ after: _____

Challenges: _____

Max effort/breathing/pulse: _____

Core: _____

Stretching: _____

Successes: _____

Other: _____

Time/Distance/Totals, if any: _____

22

Date, day, time, location: _____

Feeling of energy/health before: _____ *during:* _____ *after:* _____

Challenges: _____

Max effort/breathing/pulse: _____

Core: _____

Stretching: _____

Successes: _____

Other: _____

Time/Distance/Totals, if any: _____

23

Date, day, time, location: _____

Feeling of energy/health before: _____ *during:* _____ *after:* _____

Challenges: _____

Max effort/breathing/pulse: _____

Core: _____

Stretching: _____

Successes: _____

Other: _____

Time/Distance/Totals, if any: _____

24

Date, day, time, location: _____

Feeling of energy/health before: _____ *during:* _____ *after:* _____

Challenges: _____

Max effort/breathing/pulse: _____

Core: _____

Stretching: _____

Successes: _____

Other: _____

Time/Distance/Totals, if any: _____

25

Date, day, time, location: _____

Feeling of energy/health before: _____ *during:* _____ *after:* _____

Challenges: _____

Max effort/breathing/pulse: _____

Core: _____

Stretching: _____

Successes: _____

Other: _____

Time/Distance/Totals, if any: _____

26

Date, day, time, location: _____

Feeling of energy/health before: _____ *during:* _____ *after:* _____

Challenges: _____

Max effort/breathing/pulse: _____

Core: _____

Stretching: _____

Successes: _____

Other: _____

Time/Distance/Totals, if any: _____

27

Date, day, time, location: _____

Feeling of energy/health before: _____ *during:* _____ *after:* _____

Challenges: _____

Max effort/breathing/pulse: _____

Core: _____

Stretching: _____

Successes: _____

Other: _____

Time/Distance/Totals, if any: _____

28

Date, day, time, location: _____

Feeling of energy/health before: _____ *during:* _____ *after:* _____

Challenges: _____

Max effort/breathing/pulse: _____

Core: _____

Stretching: _____

Successes: _____

Other: _____

Time/Distance/Totals, if any: _____

29

Date, day, time, location: _____

Feeling of energy/health before: _____during:_____ after: _____

Challenges: _____

Max effort/breathing/pulse: _____

Core: _____

Stretching: _____

Successes: _____

Other: _____

Time/Distance/Totals, if any: _____

30

Date, day, time, location: _____

Feeling of energy/health before: _____during:_____ after: _____

Challenges: _____

Max effort/breathing/pulse: _____

Core: _____

Stretching: _____

Successes: _____

Other: _____

Time/Distance/Totals, if any: _____

31

Date, day, time, location: _____

Feeling of energy/health before: _____during:_____ after: _____

Challenges: _____

Max effort/breathing/pulse: _____

Core: _____

Stretching: _____

Successes: _____

Other: _____

Time/Distance/Totals, if any: _____

Extra Workouts 1
Date, day, time, location: _____
Feeling of energy/health before: _____ *during:* _____ *after:* _____
Challenges: _____
Max effort/breathing/pulse: _____
Core: _____
Stretching: _____
Successes: _____
Other: _____
Time/Distance/Totals, if any: _____

Extra 2
Date, day, time, location: _____
Feeling of energy/health before: _____ *during:* _____ *after:* _____
Challenges: _____
Max effort/breathing/pulse: _____
Core: _____
Stretching: _____
Successes: _____
Other: _____
Time/Distance/Totals, if any: _____

Extra 3
Date, day, time, location: _____
Feeling of energy/health before: _____ *during:* _____ *after:* _____
Challenges: _____
Max effort/breathing/pulse: _____
Core: _____
Stretching: _____
Successes: _____
Other: _____
Time/Distance/Totals, if any: _____

Extra 4
Date, day, time, location: _____
Feeling of energy/health before: _____ *during:* _____ *after:* _____
Challenges: _____
Max effort/breathing/pulse: _____
Core: _____

Stretching: _____

Successes: _____

Other: _____

Time/Distance/Totals, if any: _____

Extra 5

Date, day, time, location: _____

Feeling of energy/health before: _____during:_____ after: _____

Challenges: _____

Max effort/breathing/pulse: _____

Core: _____

Stretching: _____

Successes: _____

Other: _____

Time/Distance/Totals, if any: _____

End of Month Scoring

Method One: Basic (Number of days I exercised this month): _____
    Ultimate Goal: Every Day
    My Goal for This Month Was: _____
    My Goal for Next Month Is: _____
Method Two: Subtraction (Days I Rowed Minus Days Not): _____
    Initial Goal: Exceed Zero (row at least half the days)
    Ultimate Goal: Same as days in the month.
    My Goal for This Month Was: _____
    My Goal for Next Month Is: _____
Method Three: Division (Percentage = Days Rowed Divided by Total Days): _____
    Ultimate Goal: 100%
    My Goal for This Month Was: _____
    My Goal for Next Month Is: _____

Other Scores and Data for Month (Goals set and met; Times rowed; Distances rowed; Other):

_____

_____

_____

_____

_____

_____

_____

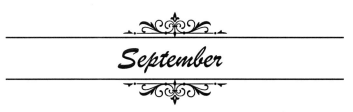

September

"When coupled, inactivity and aging seem to accelerate the effects of aging. . . . Because inactivity appears to accelerate the aging process, the progressive loss of tissues of muscles, nerves, and various vital organs may be delayed . . . by participation in a regular exercise program. The proverbial wisdom 'use it or lose it' is especially pertinent for the elderly."
　　Encyclopedia, at 595-96

"If the man who wrote the Declaration of Independence, was Secretary of State, and twice President, could give it two hours, our children can give it ten or fifteen minutes."
　　John F. Kennedy (12/5/61 address)

"There are six components of wellness: proper weight and diet, proper exercise, breaking the smoking habit, control of alcohol, stress management and periodic exams."
　　Dr. Kenneth Cooper

"Cardiac patients by their very nature tend to be sedentary. It's important to tell them you don't have to be a marathon runner. What we are asking for is really very mild levels of activity, but they need to occur pretty often, thirty minutes a day for at least three days a week."
　　Dr. Michael Lauer, Kolata, at 67

"Why do we breathe? . . . Breath, as we all know, is life, an equivalence that's been recognized all over the world for thousands of years. For example, remember that the [Sanskrit] word prana is rooted in the verb an, which means 'to breathe,' but also 'to live' and 'to move.'"
　　Richard Rosen, The Yoga of Breath, A Step-by-Step Guide to Pranayama, at 21

"Specifically, exercise can do the following:
- Make the heart stronger. . . .
- Improve circulation. . . .
- Decrease blood pressure.
- Decrease . . . cholesterol . . . .
- Make muscles stronger and increase flexibility. . . .
- Make bones denser and stronger. . . .

[and the list goes on with more than a dozen additional benefits]."
　　Merck, at 806-07

September – Fall Rowing, Fall Racing and the Aerobic Base

Not too many generations ago, rowing was considered a seasonal sport. The high school and college racing season was the spring and, at least on some teams, you could do other sports in other seasons. Then, when you showed up at the boathouse in late winter, you might still get in a boat that spring. Amazingly, some high school programs even today still regard the sport as a one-season activity and regulate it as such. And let's not get into NCAA restrictions on collegiate rowing, which seems like a medieval regulatory framework that is based on a lack of understanding of how rowers learn to row well and fast.

Even back in 1970, however, some coaches recognized that the fall was a time to build their rowers' aerobic base. It may not have been called that at the time, because Dr. Cooper's revolutionary book "Aerobics" had only come out two years before. But some rowing coaches knew from their own experience that there were positive effects available through more regular year-round training. Fall distance rowing would give a team a stronger foundation for intense spring sprint races. And, as United States coaches began to learn that a higher level of fitness was possible through year-round training, the longer rows of autumn became even more standard.

At that time, fall racing was relatively new, infrequent and informal. In the ensuing 40 years, it has become perhaps the most active racing season in rowing in terms of number of participants, with large-scale head races occurring all over from September to October or November (depending to some degree on local climate).

Whether you race or not, September is a great time to focus on longer rows.

If you have been doing short, intense pieces (whether racing others informally or just on your own) during the summer, ratchet your pace back slightly and see what you can do for a longer piece. If you find you want to stop as you increase your distance, instead ease up the pressure a little and/or take the stroke down a bit, and try to keep going. Both long term fitness gains and fat-burning effects can be substantial from long rows even at paces substantially slower than your peak pace.

On a rowing machine, you can set the time or distance you will row and moderate your pace according to how you feel. On the water, you can plan on rowing to a more distant point or doing an extra lap if you are on a small lake.

Using either medium, look for a training benefit as well as a fitness benefit. In terms of your fitness, you will discover eventually that, as a result of doing more long rows, you can maintain a faster pace for a longer time or distance than you used to be able to do. And as a training benefit, you will find that by rowing longer you will eventually relax more. Relaxing more while still rowing with firm pressure can result in a natural improvement in your technique. Sometimes it is the 8th or 9th or 10th mile when you are tired and on your way back to the boathouse (or to the end of the indoor row) that your body loses the unnecessary extra motions, your posture improves and your efficiency rises, with the result that you go faster while feeling more comfortable. Rowing should look easy. With longer rows, your rowing likely will begin to look more relaxed and feel better even as it becomes stronger.

Ron looks forward to racing every fall. From head races near where he lives to one or more of the national and international favorites, he usually competes several times and has medaled on many occasions in his age group.

Mel did not race during the summer but got out in a single and is thinking about racing in the fall next year. That will give her time to work on her technique and fitness.

Andie is volunteering at a major fall regatta to learn more about how they are run, watch the races and meet other rowers. She figures that if her rowing vacation works out next year, she might compete in the fall.

What shall I do today . . . heute . . . hoy . . . aujourd'hui . . . oggi . . . idag . . . tanaan . . . avui . . .

1

Date, day, time, location: _____

Feeling of energy/health before: _____during:_____ after: _____

Challenges: _____

Max effort/breathing/pulse: _____

Core: _____

Stretching: _____

Successes: _____

Other: _____

Time/Distance/Totals, if any: _____

2

Date, day, time, location: _____

Feeling of energy/health before: _____during:_____ after: _____

Challenges: _____

Max effort/breathing/pulse: _____

Core: _____

Stretching: _____

Successes: _____

Other: _____

Time/Distance/Totals, if any: _____

3

Date, day, time, location: _____

Feeling of energy/health before: _____during:_____ after: _____

Challenges: _____

Max effort/breathing/pulse: _____

Core: _____

Stretching: _____

Successes: _____

Other: _____

Time/Distance/Totals, if any: _____

4

Date, day, time, location: _____

Feeling of energy/health before: _____during:_____ after: _____

Challenges: _____

Max effort/breathing/pulse: _____

Core: _____

Stretching: _____

Successes: _____

Other: _____

Time/Distance/Totals, if any: _____

5

Date, day, time, location: _____

Feeling of energy/health before: _____ *during:* _____ *after:* _____

Challenges: _____

Max effort/breathing/pulse: _____

Core: _____

Stretching: _____

Successes: _____

Other: _____

Time/Distance/Totals, if any: _____

6

Date, day, time, location: _____

Feeling of energy/health before: _____ *during:* _____ *after:* _____

Challenges: _____

Max effort/breathing/pulse: _____

Core: _____

Stretching: _____

Successes: _____

Other: _____

Time/Distance/Totals, if any: _____

7

Date, day, time, location: _____

Feeling of energy/health before: _____ *during:* _____ *after:* _____

Challenges: _____

Max effort/breathing/pulse: _____

Core: _____

Stretching: _____

Successes: _____

Other: _____

Time/Distance/Totals, if any: _____

8

Date, day, time, location: _____

Feeling of energy/health before: _____*during:*_____ *after:* _____

Challenges: _____

Max effort/breathing/pulse: _____

Core: _____

Stretching: _____

Successes: _____

Other: _____

Time/Distance/Totals, if any: _____

9

Date, day, time, location: _____

Feeling of energy/health before: _____*during:*_____ *after:* _____

Challenges: _____

Max effort/breathing/pulse: _____

Core: _____

Stretching: _____

Successes: _____

Other: _____

Time/Distance/Totals, if any: _____

10

Date, day, time, location: _____

Feeling of energy/health before: _____*during:*_____ *after:* _____

Challenges: _____

Max effort/breathing/pulse: _____

Core: _____

Stretching: _____

Successes: _____

Other: _____

Time/Distance/Totals, if any: _____

11

Date, day, time, location: _____

Feeling of energy/health before: _____*during:*_____ *after:* _____

Challenges: _____

Max effort/breathing/pulse: _____

Core: _____

Stretching: _____

Successes: _____

Other: _____

Time/Distance/Totals, if any: _____

12

Date, day, time, location: _____

Feeling of energy/health before: _____during:_____ after: _____

Challenges: _____

Max effort/breathing/pulse: _____

Core: _____

Stretching: _____

Successes: _____

Other: _____

Time/Distance/Totals, if any: _____

13

Date, day, time, location: _____

Feeling of energy/health before: _____during:_____ after: _____

Challenges: _____ _____

Max effort/breathing/pulse: _____

Core: _____

Stretching: _____

Successes: _____

Other: _____

Time/Distance/Totals, if any: _____

14

Date, day, time, location: _____

Feeling of energy/health before: _____during:_____ after: _____

Challenges: _____

Max effort/breathing/pulse: _____

Core: _____

Stretching: _____

Successes: _____

Other: _____

Time/Distance/Totals, if any: _____

15

Date, day, time, location: _____

Feeling of energy/health before: _____ *during:* _____ *after:* _____

Challenges: _____

Max effort/breathing/pulse: _____

Core: _____

Stretching: _____

Successes: _____

Other: _____

Time/Distance/Totals, if any: _____

16

Date, day, time, location: _____

Feeling of energy/health before: _____ *during:* _____ *after:* _____

Challenges: _____

Max effort/breathing/pulse: _____

Core: _____

Stretching: _____

Successes: _____

Other: _____

Time/Distance/Totals, if any: _____

17

Date, day, time, location: _____

Feeling of energy/health before: _____ *during:* _____ *after:* _____

Challenges: _____

Max effort/breathing/pulse: _____

Core: _____

Stretching: _____

Successes: _____

Other: _____

Time/Distance/Totals, if any: _____

18

Date, day, time, location: _____

Feeling of energy/health before: _____ *during:* _____ *after:* _____

Challenges: _____

Max effort/breathing/pulse: _____

Core: _____

Stretching: _____

Successes: _____

Other: _____

Time/Distance/Totals, if any: _____

19

Date, day, time, location: _____

Feeling of energy/health before: _____during:_____ after: _____

Challenges: _____

Max effort/breathing/pulse: _____

Core: _____

Stretching: _____

Successes: _____

Other: _____

Time/Distance/Totals, if any: _____

20

Date, day, time, location: _____

Feeling of energy/health before: _____during:_____ after: _____

Challenges: _____

Max effort/breathing/pulse: _____

Core: _____

Stretching: _____

Successes: _____

Other: _____

Time/Distance/Totals, if any: _____

21

Date, day, time, location: _____

Feeling of energy/health before: _____during:_____ after: _____

Challenges: _____

Max effort/breathing/pulse: _____

Core: _____

Stretching: _____

Successes: _____

Other: _____

Time/Distance/Totals, if any: _____

22

Date, day, time, location: _____

Feeling of energy/health before: _____*during:*_____ *after:* _____

Challenges: _____

Max effort/breathing/pulse: _____

Core: _____

Stretching: _____

Successes: _____

Other: _____

Time/Distance/Totals, if any: _____

23

Date, day, time, location: _____

Feeling of energy/health before: _____*during:*_____ *after:* _____

Challenges: _____

Max effort/breathing/pulse: _____

Core: _____

Stretching: _____

Successes: _____

Other: _____

Time/Distance/Totals, if any: _____

24

Date, day, time, location: _____

Feeling of energy/health before: _____*during:*_____ *after:* _____

Challenges: _____

Max effort/breathing/pulse: _____

Core: _____

Stretching: _____

Successes: _____

Other: _____

Time/Distance/Totals, if any: _____

25

Date, day, time, location: _____

Feeling of energy/health before: _____*during:*_____ *after:* _____

Challenges: _____

Max effort/breathing/pulse: _____

Core: _____

Stretching: _____

Successes: _____

Other: _____

Time/Distance/Totals, if any: _____

26

Date, day, time, location: _____

Feeling of energy/health before: _____*during:*_____ *after:* _____

Challenges: _____

Max effort/breathing/pulse: _____

Core: _____

Stretching: _____

Successes: _____

Other: _____

Time/Distance/Totals, if any: _____

27

Date, day, time, location: _____

Feeling of energy/health before: _____*during:*_____ *after:* _____

Challenges: _____

Max effort/breathing/pulse: _____

Core: _____

Stretching: _____

Successes: _____

Other: _____

Time/Distance/Totals, if any: _____

28

Date, day, time, location: _____

Feeling of energy/health before: _____*during:*_____ *after:* _____

Challenges: _____

Max effort/breathing/pulse: _____

Core: _____

Stretching: _____

Successes: _____

Other: _____

Time/Distance/Totals, if any: _____

29

Date, day, time, location: _____

Feeling of energy/health before: _____ *during:* _____ *after:* _____

Challenges: _____

Max effort/breathing/pulse: _____

Core: _____

Stretching: _____

Successes: _____

Other: _____

Time/Distance/Totals, if any: _____

30

Date, day, time, location: _____

Feeling of energy/health before: _____ *during:* _____ *after:* _____

Challenges: _____

Max effort/breathing/pulse: _____

Core: _____

Stretching: _____

Successes: _____

Other: _____

Time/Distance/Totals, if any: _____

31

Date, day, time, location: _____

Feeling of energy/health before: _____ *during:* _____ *after:* _____

Challenges: _____

Max effort/breathing/pulse: _____

Core: _____

Stretching: _____

Successes: _____

Other: _____

Time/Distance/Totals, if any: _____

Extra Workouts 1
Date, day, time, location: _____
Feeling of energy/health before: _____during:_____ after: _____
Challenges: _____
Max effort/breathing/pulse: _____
Core: _____
Stretching: _____
Successes: _____
Other: _____
Time/Distance/Totals, if any: _____

Extra 2
Date, day, time, location: _____
Feeling of energy/health before: _____during:_____ after: _____
Challenges: _____
Max effort/breathing/pulse: _____
Core: _____
Stretching: _____
Successes: _____
Other: _____
Time/Distance/Totals, if any: _____

Extra 3
Date, day, time, location: _____
Feeling of energy/health before: _____during:_____ after: _____
Challenges: _____
Max effort/breathing/pulse: _____
Core: _____
Stretching: _____
Successes: _____
Other: _____
Time/Distance/Totals, if any: _____

Extra 4
Date, day, time, location: _____
Feeling of energy/health before: _____during:_____ after: _____
Challenges: _____
Max effort/breathing/pulse: _____
Core: _____

What shall I do today . . . heute . . . hoy . . . aujourd'hui . . . oggi . . . idag . . . tanaan . . . avui . . .

Stretching: _____

Successes: _____

Other: _____

Time/Distance/Totals, if any: _____

Extra 5

Date, day, time, location: _____

Feeling of energy/health before: _____*during:*_____ *after:* _____

Challenges: _____

Max effort/breathing/pulse: _____

Core: _____

Stretching: _____

Successes: _____

Other: _____

Time/Distance/Totals, if any: _____

End of Month Scoring

Method One: Basic (Number of days I exercised this month):_____
    Ultimate Goal: Every Day
    My Goal for This Month Was: _____
    My Goal for Next Month Is: _____
Method Two: Subtraction (Days I Rowed Minus Days Not):_____
    Initial Goal: Exceed Zero (row at least half the days)
    Ultimate Goal: Same as days in the month.
    My Goal for This Month Was: _____
    My Goal for Next Month Is: _____
Method Three: Division (Percentage = Days Rowed Divided by Total Days): _____
    Ultimate Goal: 100%
    My Goal for This Month Was:_____
    My Goal for Next Month Is: _____

Other Scores and Data for Month (Goals set and met; Times rowed; Distances rowed; Other):

_____

_____

_____

_____

_____

_____

Season Recap and Change

Scoring

You have calculated your score at the end of each month. Take a season-long look at your progress. Where have you improved during the three months of this season? Compare season to season as the year progresses. Most importantly, once you calculate your score, consider whether it correlates with how you feel.

_____

_____

_____

_____

_____

Goals Accomplished

Look back on your goals for the past season. Did you set goals for your score based on how many days you rowed? Did you set goals to row longer each day? If you are succeeding with both of those challenges, how are you doing at including core work and stretching each day? (Are you recording that?) Do you also set goals for distances rowed or pace? Have you planned to take a rowing class or attend a rowing event? For these and other goals you may have set three months ago, look back and record here how you did.

_____

_____

_____

_____

_____

_____

Goals Looking Ahead

Once you have looked back, plan ahead. Set some goals. Make them realistic based on your past experience, events coming up and your other plans for the coming three months.

_____

_____

_____

_____

_____

Changes for Variety

Do you cross-train for variety? How can you modify that in the coming season? Plan a vacation based on doing something active you would enjoy. Add an aerobics or spinning or Pilates class or some weight lifting or yoga or something else you may not normally do.

_____

_____

_____

_____

_____

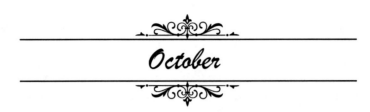

October

"If you don't do what's best for your body, you're the one who comes up on the short end."
  Julius Erving

"Exercise helps alleviate age-related changes in sleep patterns, and appears to reduce anxiety and promote a sense of well-being. Regular exercise may also play a role in the rate of deterioration of sense organ function."
  Encyclopedia, at 587

"By the middle of the nineteenth century, American doctors were sounding a surprisingly modern cry of despair. With changing lifestyles . . ., the population was becoming sedentary. They simply had to get more exercise, doctors said."
  Kolata, at 36

"Most middle-aged adults who exercise regularly will be healthier in later years . . . . A person endowed with few risk factors may experience only a small boost in life expectancy. However, for a person with numerous inherited risk factors, like coronary artery disease and high blood pressure, exercise can dramatically improve life expectancy."
  Encyclopedia, at 600

"Do your own thing, as long as it raises your heart level to more than 120 beats a minute for half an hour—four times a week."
  George Sheehan, Kolata, at 47

"Regular exercise can reduce many of the effects of aging on the heart and blood vessels."
  Merck, at 15

"Exercise does not have to involve working up a drenching sweat. Moderate exercise, preferably every day, provides significant health benefits. The key is doing moderately active things regularly."
  Merck, at 806

October – Transition to Indoor Rowing

At some point in the fall, if you have been rowing outdoors, you likely will prepare to transition to indoor rowing for a season or two. Even in a warmer climate, many rowers use the change of seasons to modify their exercise routine as fall racing ends. They may still row outdoors some of the time through the winter, but likely will intersperse their outdoors rows with indoor rowing, weight lifting and other forms of complementary exercise.

If you are in a northern climate, you will likely have to walk through frost on the dock before your morning row more than once before you put your shell away for the winter and shift to indoor rowing. There is nothing like those barefoot imprints in an early frost on the dock to tell you the seasons are changing. As the years pass, you may find you are more and more averse to feeling cold. At the same time, knowing how much you will want to get back on the water in the spring after months exercising indoors (or skiing and doing other winter activities to cross-train) may strengthen your resolve to put up with the challenges of late fall rowing. Adjust your rowing times if you can to use the daylight. Get lights for your boat if you must start or finish in the dark. Know the safety rules of your lake or river. Row with a partner for safety.

As you shift to indoor rowing, think about your goals for the winter and spring and consider what you can do to achieve them. Ask yourself what your weak points are and incorporate something early on to address those.

- If you had an enjoyable summer rowing but feel weak, gear your indoor rowing and cross-training to increase your strength. Incorporate different interval work and add some weight lifting.
- If you feel worn out from an intense season of racing, consider whether you are ready to begin training right away for races several months away, or you want some relief. One of the hardest things for a competing rower to do is to row lightly or easily, but consider some low stroke work to rest while maintaining or even improving your basic aerobic fitness.
- If you feel strong but undirected, consider winter, spring and summer races you might want to plan for as a target to give yourself a goal and to lend some direction to your training.
- If you are just beginning or going back indoors for the first time, simply work out a schedule to follow. Getting into the groove of regular rows on the machine may be more important for you than what you do on a given day.

And if you are rowing comfortably for health and have no plans to race or to set such goals, use the change of seasons to review what you have done and to spice up your workout routine.

Consider your goals for the coming month and quarter. Look back at your training success in terms of days rowed per month and consider planning to improve on it. Look ahead to indoor rowing challenges and races and consider making one your goal. You can row an indoor race for the experience even if you know your time will not make you competitive with the winners for your age group. Setting the goal to race will give you another incentive to row regularly. Participating will teach you something about how the body works, from the power of adrenaline in the first strokes to various lessons throughout the race. And, even if you deliberately race at a pace you know you can comfortably maintain without the stress or pain of pushing your limits, that experience also is useful and can be enjoyable.

The holiday season is both a problem and an incentive to train more. With parties and other events coming up in the last two months of the calendar year, it may be harder than usual to get in your daily row. And it is easier to put on weight, to slow down, to feel like you are entering hibernation. But look at it as a challenge, a reason to row longer when you can and to find ways to get in more rows per week. Your fitness may be a small part of your destiny, but it is one we can each control to some degree. See what you can do to get through the end of the year successfully.

Ron evaluates his past racing results and future competition plans at this time of year and tweaks his routine for the coming year. And he starts up the process of focusing his training on the races he wants to compete in the following summer and fall.

Mel is looking forward to indoor rowing with a different set of expectations than she had last year. Now, she is a rower. She may be a beginning rower, but she knows enough to train on her own, who to go to for guidance or encouragement, when she can take classes, and more. She does not plan out a month-to-month regimen for herself, but she has ideas and goals, and that makes it easier for her to row each day.

Andie is looking into fitness classes she can use to complement her indoor rowing. She is thinking of going to one of the indoor rowing races in February to see how she can do, and is starting to experiment with a weekly routine of variable steady state and interval training rows.

1

Date, day, time, location: _____

Feeling of energy/health before: _____during:_____ after: _____

Challenges: _____

Max effort/breathing/pulse: _____

Core: _____

Stretching: _____

Successes: _____

Other: _____

Time/Distance/Totals, if any: _____

2

Date, day, time, location: _____

Feeling of energy/health before: _____during:_____ after: _____

Challenges: _____

Max effort/breathing/pulse: _____

Core: _____

Stretching: _____

Successes: _____

Other: _____

Time/Distance/Totals, if any: _____

3

Date, day, time, location: _____

Feeling of energy/health before: _____during:_____ after: _____

Challenges: _____

Max effort/breathing/pulse: _____

Core: _____

Stretching: _____

Successes: _____

Other: _____

Time/Distance/Totals, if any: _____

4

Date, day, time, location: _____

Feeling of energy/health before: _____during:_____ after: _____

Challenges: _____

Max effort/breathing/pulse: _____

Core: _____

What shall I do today . . . heute . . . hoy . . . aujourd'hui . . . oggi . . . idag . . . tanaan . . . avui . . .

Stretching: _____

Successes: _____

Other: _____

Time/Distance/Totals, if any: _____

5

Date, day, time, location: _____

Feeling of energy/health before: _____ *during:* _____ *after:* _____

Challenges: _____

Max effort/breathing/pulse: _____

Core: _____

Stretching: _____

Successes: _____

Other: _____

Time/Distance/Totals, if any: _____

6

Date, day, time, location: _____

Feeling of energy/health before: _____ *during:* _____ *after:* _____

Challenges: _____

Max effort/breathing/pulse: _____

Core: _____

Stretching: _____

Successes: _____

Other: _____

Time/Distance/Totals, if any: _____

7

Date, day, time, location: _____

Feeling of energy/health before: _____ *during:* _____ *after:* _____

Challenges: _____

Max effort/breathing/pulse: _____

Core: _____

Stretching: _____

Successes: _____

Other: _____

Time/Distance/Totals, if any: _____

8

Date, day, time, location: _____

Feeling of energy/health before: _____*during:*_____ *after:* _____

Challenges: _____

Max effort/breathing/pulse: _____

Core: _____

Stretching: _____

Successes: _____

Other: _____

Time/Distance/Totals, if any: _____

9

Date, day, time, location: _____

Feeling of energy/health before: _____*during:*_____ *after:* _____

Challenges: _____

Max effort/breathing/pulse: _____

Core: _____

Stretching: _____

Successes: _____

Other: _____

Time/Distance/Totals, if any: _____

10

Date, day, time, location: _____

Feeling of energy/health before: _____*during:*_____ *after:* _____

Challenges: _____

Max effort/breathing/pulse: _____

Core: _____

Stretching: _____

Successes: _____

Other: _____

Time/Distance/Totals, if any: _____

11

Date, day, time, location: _____

Feeling of energy/health before: _____*during:*_____ *after:* _____

Challenges: _____

Max effort/breathing/pulse: _____

Core: _____

What shall I do today . . . heute . . . hoy . . . aujourd'hui . . . oggi . . . idag . . . tanaan . . . avui . . .

Stretching: _____

Successes: _____

Other: _____

Time/Distance/Totals, if any: _____

12

Date, day, time, location: _____

Feeling of energy/health before: _____ *during:* _____ *after:* _____

Challenges: _____

Max effort/breathing/pulse: _____

Core: _____

Stretching: _____

Successes: _____

Other: _____

Time/Distance/Totals, if any: _____

13

Date, day, time, location: _____

Feeling of energy/health before: _____ *during:* _____ *after:* _____

Challenges: _____

Max effort/breathing/pulse: _____

Core: _____

Stretching: _____

Successes: _____

Other: _____

Time/Distance/Totals, if any: _____

14

Date, day, time, location: _____

Feeling of energy/health before: _____ *during:* _____ *after:* _____

Challenges: _____

Max effort/breathing/pulse: _____

Core: _____

Stretching: _____

Successes: _____

Other: _____

Time/Distance/Totals, if any: _____

15

Date, day, time, location: _____

Feeling of energy/health before: _____*during:*_____ *after:* _____

Challenges: _____

Max effort/breathing/pulse: _____

Core: _____

Stretching: _____

Successes: _____

Other: _____

Time/Distance/Totals, if any: _____

16

Date, day, time, location: _____

Feeling of energy/health before: _____*during:*_____ *after:* _____

Challenges: _____

Max effort/breathing/pulse: _____

Core: _____

Stretching: _____

Successes: _____

Other: _____

Time/Distance/Totals, if any: _____

17

Date, day, time, location: _____

Feeling of energy/health before: _____*during:*_____ *after:* _____

Challenges: _____

Max effort/breathing/pulse: _____

Core: _____

Stretching: _____

Successes: _____

Other: _____

Time/Distance/Totals, if any: _____

18

Date, day, time, location: _____

Feeling of energy/health before: _____*during:*_____ *after:* _____

Challenges: _____

Max effort/breathing/pulse: _____

Core: _____

What shall I do today . . . heute . . . hoy . . . aujourd'hui . . . oggi . . . idag . . . tanaan . . . avui . . .

Stretching: _____

Successes: _____

Other: _____

Time/Distance/Totals, if any: _____

19

Date, day, time, location: _____

Feeling of energy/health before: _____ *during:* _____ *after:* _____

Challenges: _____

Max effort/breathing/pulse: _____

Core: _____

Stretching: _____

Successes: _____

Other: _____

Time/Distance/Totals, if any: _____

20

Date, day, time, location: _____

Feeling of energy/health before: _____ *during:* _____ *after:* _____

Challenges: _____

Max effort/breathing/pulse: _____

Core: _____

Stretching: _____

Successes: _____

Other: _____

Time/Distance/Totals, if any: _____

21

Date, day, time, location: _____

Feeling of energy/health before: _____ *during:* _____ *after:* _____

Challenges: _____

Max effort/breathing/pulse: _____

Core: _____

Stretching: _____

Successes: _____

Other: _____

Time/Distance/Totals, if any: _____

22

Date, day, time, location: _____

Feeling of energy/health before: _____*during:*_____ *after:* _____

Challenges: _____

Max effort/breathing/pulse: _____

Core: _____

Stretching: _____

Successes: _____

Other: _____

Time/Distance/Totals, if any: _____

23

Date, day, time, location: _____

Feeling of energy/health before: _____*during:*_____ *after:* _____

Challenges: _____

Max effort/breathing/pulse: _____

Core: _____

Stretching: _____

Successes: _____

Other: _____

Time/Distance/Totals, if any: _____

24

Date, day, time, location: _____

Feeling of energy/health before: _____*during:*_____ *after:* _____

Challenges: _____

Max effort/breathing/pulse: _____

Core: _____

Stretching: _____

Successes: _____

Other: _____

Time/Distance/Totals, if any: _____

25

Date, day, time, location: _____

Feeling of energy/health before: _____*during:*_____ *after:* _____

Challenges: _____

Max effort/breathing/pulse: _____

Core: _____

What shall I do today . . . heute . . . hoy . . . aujourd'hui . . . oggi . . . idag . . . tanaan . . . avui . . .

Stretching: _____

Successes: _____

Other: _____

Time/Distance/Totals, if any: _____

26

Date, day, time, location: _____

Feeling of energy/health before: _____ *during:* _____ *after:* _____

Challenges: _____

Max effort/breathing/pulse: _____

Core: _____

Stretching: _____

Successes: _____

Other: _____

Time/Distance/Totals, if any: _____

27

Date, day, time, location: _____

Feeling of energy/health before: _____ *during:* _____ *after:* _____

Challenges: _____

Max effort/breathing/pulse: _____

Core: _____

Stretching: _____

Successes: _____

Other: _____

Time/Distance/Totals, if any: _____

28

Date, day, time, location: _____

Feeling of energy/health before: _____ *during:* _____ *after:* _____

Challenges: _____

Max effort/breathing/pulse: _____

Core: _____

Stretching: _____

Successes: _____

Other: _____

Time/Distance/Totals, if any: _____

29

Date, day, time, location: _____

Feeling of energy/health before: _____during:_____ after: _____

Challenges: _____

Max effort/breathing/pulse: _____

Core: _____

Stretching: _____

Successes: _____

Other: _____

Time/Distance/Totals, if any: _____

30

Date, day, time, location: _____

Feeling of energy/health before: _____during:_____ after: _____

Challenges: _____

Max effort/breathing/pulse: _____

Core: _____

Stretching: _____

Successes: _____

Other: _____

Time/Distance/Totals, if any: _____

31

Date, day, time, location: _____

Feeling of energy/health before: _____during:_____ after: _____

Challenges: _____

Max effort/breathing/pulse: _____

Core: _____

Stretching: _____

Successes: _____

Other: _____

Time/Distance/Totals, if any: _____

Extra Workouts 1

Date, day, time, location: _____

Feeling of energy/health before: _____*during:*_____ *after:* _____

Challenges: _____

Max effort/breathing/pulse: _____

Core: _____

Stretching: _____

Successes: _____

Other: _____

Time/Distance/Totals, if any: _____

Extra 2

Date, day, time, location: _____

Feeling of energy/health before: _____*during:*_____ *after:* _____

Challenges: _____

Max effort/breathing/pulse: _____

Core: _____

Stretching: _____

Successes: _____

Other: _____

Time/Distance/Totals, if any: _____

Extra 3

Date, day, time, location: _____

Feeling of energy/health before: _____*during:*_____ *after:* _____

Challenges: _____

Max effort/breathing/pulse: _____

Core: _____

Stretching: _____

Successes: _____

Other: _____

Time/Distance/Totals, if any: _____

Extra 4

Date, day, time, location: _____

Feeling of energy/health before: _____*during:*_____ *after:* _____

Challenges: _____

Max effort/breathing/pulse: _____

Core: _____

Stretching: _____

Successes: _____

Other: _____

Time/Distance/Totals, if any: _____

Extra 5

Date, day, time, location: _____

Feeling of energy/health before: _____*during:*_____ *after:* _____

Challenges: _____

Max effort/breathing/pulse: _____

Core: _____

Stretching: _____

Successes: _____

Other: _____

Time/Distance/Totals, if any: _____

What shall I do today . . . heute . . . hoy . . . aujourd'hui . . . oggi . . . idag . . . tanaan . . . avui . . .

End of Month Scoring

Method One: Basic (Number of days I exercised this month):_____
    Ultimate Goal: Every Day
    My Goal for This Month Was: _____
    My Goal for Next Month Is: _____
Method Two: Subtraction (Days I Rowed Minus Days Not):_____
    Initial Goal: Exceed Zero (row at least half the days)
    Ultimate Goal: Same as days in the month.
    My Goal for This Month Was: _____
    My Goal for Next Month Is: _____
Method Three: Division (Percentage = Days Rowed Divided by Total Days): _____
    Ultimate Goal: 100%
    My Goal for This Month Was:_____
    My Goal for Next Month Is: _____

Other Scores and Data for Month (Goals set and met; Times rowed; Distances rowed; Other):

_____

_____

_____

_____

_____

_____

_____

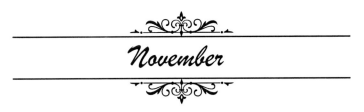

November

"My parents always wanted me to be above average, but this [exercise] is one area where average is fine."
  Michael Lauer, MD

"Time and again, when I ask people why they keep exercising, year in and year out, they tell me that they started exercising to lose weight, or to help their hearts, or to firm up their bodies, and kept at it because they discovered that they loved physical exertion."
  Kolata, at 266

"Physical fitness is not only one of the most important keys to a healthy body; it is the basis of dynamic and creative intellectual activity."
  John F. Kennedy

"Regular exercise may help in maintaining a positive self-image and attitude because it generates feelings of endurance, strength, and vitality.
  Encyclopedia, at 585

"Regular exercise can partially overcome or at least significantly delay the loss of muscle mass and strength [that comes with aging]. . . . [E]ven people who have never exercised can increase muscle mass and strength."
  Merck, at 13

"Regular weight-bearing exercise plays a major role in retarding the loss of bone mass."
  Encyclopedia, at 586

November – Weightlifting

Weightlifting is an exceptionally useful method of cross-training for rowers. Rowing involves a rare combination of strength and endurance. Because of the duration of most rowing practices and races (other than a sprint race), it is mostly aerobic and supports the cardio-vascular development of the entire body. At the same time, rowers move more slowly (30 strokes per minute) than, say, a cyclist or spinner, whose legs will repeat their motion many more times per minute. The strength component in rowing is therefore more pronounced. Weight lifting can help develop a rower, help bring her to a higher level, by using fewer muscles for fewer repetitions in each lift in a way that stimulates increased strength she can then use when she rows.

As a rule, take a lesson in safe weight lifting before you start to lift on your own if you are not an experienced weight lifter. Be sure you know what you are doing and you are in a safe environment. Do not overdo it, especially when first adding a weightlifting routine to your regimen. If you are lifting heavy weight (for you; keep in mind that is a subjective, personal standard), be sure you have a spotter.

Use free weights (rather than weight machines) as your method of preference if you have both available. Free weights allow your body to work on balance and coordination while you lift. But there is no harm in also using machines on which you sit down and work limited portions of the body as a secondary weight lifting method.

Select a small number of weight lifting exercises, perhaps three or four, to begin unless you have a full routine a friend or coach has provided which you can follow. For example, you could try a squat, a curl, a press and one other exercise of your choice. Unless you have been trained in a lengthy routine including many lifts, keep it simple and focused. For example, if a trainer or someone with more experience gives you a routine with a dozen lifts, they will probably explain to you how to alternate parts of the body (muscle groups) that you stimulate with the weights.

When you begin, start with a weight that is light, a weight you know you can easily move through the required motion without strain. Do so for at least one set of 5-10 repetitions (reps) simply to get used to the motion. With a curl, that is pretty basic, but with a squat, you may find that even though we all sit down and get up every day, the controlled range of motion seems to use muscles you are not used to using.

Increase the weight slightly for a second set and repeat that cycle to complete three sets, taking a minute or longer break between sets. If you are a beginner or simply out of shape, you should watch for unintended effects, issues of balance, control of the weights and so on.

What do you experience the first day (perhaps the first several days/times) you begin to acclimate your body to weight lifting? One thing you likely will notice is that the demand of lifting with some muscles results in your tightening other muscles. For example, you do a squat with a bar across your shoulders. Your back is erect and relaxed and you are using your quads, hamstrings and glutes. But you may feel like your back and other core muscles tighten, too. You may feel like your breathing is affected and even find yourself holding your breath. You may feel your arms and shoulders tensing up. You may find specific portions of the hamstrings tighten, as if they had been dormant and are now being called into service. That may call for extra stretching while other portions of the bands of muscle surrounding the legs do not seem to be so affected. Your joints may feel different, weak or uncomfortable at first. Keep the weight low and easily managed and watch how they strengthen and become more comfortable over time.

The next week or the week after that, these effects may lessen and be replaced by entirely different responses. What you will enjoy is that, while you begin to firm up the muscles you are using, you will also find over a period of weeks that these side issues go away. Your body adjusts and you get past them. Not only does your muscular strength increase, but you also will find your joints becoming more comfortable, your ability to handle more weight enhanced, and your body's ability to work hard and relax at the same time to improve.

Take it easy, skip a day between lifts of the same muscles (but that does not mean you cannot work different muscle groups on the 'off' day), and stick with your schedule - because if you skip lifting days you may have to go back a step when you start up again. The goal is to improve incrementally every time you lift with a regular routine.

Ron incorporates weight lifting every year and has a set of routines he favors for different times of year. Especially as he has aged, he has been struck with the need to lift weights just to maintain strength that, when he was younger, seemed to be a given. So, part of the way he faces that aging muscle 'wasting' challenge is with weightlifting.

Mel is not thinking of lifting weights. She knows the competitors do it. She has friends who have taken weight lifting classes and boast about their muscle tone. But she is happy with the improvements she is experiencing in her own strength and muscle tone and weight loss with her rowing. Maybe next year.

Andie is planning to lift weights three times a week during December and January, and then stop well before she races in February. She has taken a class on using free weights and instruction from her health club about using their weight machines. A friend has given her a list of six exercises to use for her upper body, legs and back.

What shall I do today . . . heute . . . hoy . . . aujourd'hui . . . oggi . . . idag . . . tanaan . . . avui . . .

1

Date, day, time, location: _____

Feeling of energy/health before: _____ *during:* _____ *after:* _____

Challenges: _____

Max effort/breathing/pulse: _____

Core: _____

Stretching: _____

Successes: _____

Other: _____

Time/Distance/Totals, if any: _____

2

Date, day, time, location: _____

Feeling of energy/health before: _____ *during:* _____ *after:* _____

Challenges: _____

Max effort/breathing/pulse: _____

Core: _____

Stretching: _____

Successes: _____

Other: _____

Time/Distance/Totals, if any: _____

3

Date, day, time, location: _____

Feeling of energy/health before: _____ *during:* _____ *after:* _____

Challenges: _____

Max effort/breathing/pulse: _____

Core: _____

Stretching: _____

Successes: _____

Other: _____

Time/Distance/Totals, if any: _____

4

Date, day, time, location: _____

Feeling of energy/health before: _____ *during:* _____ *after:* _____

Challenges: _____

Max effort/breathing/pulse: _____

Core: _____

Stretching: _____

Successes: _____

Other: _____

Time/Distance/Totals, if any: _____

5

Date, day, time, location: _____

Feeling of energy/health before: _____*during:*_____ *after:* _____

Challenges: _____

Max effort/breathing/pulse: _____

Core: _____

Stretching: _____

Successes: _____

Other: _____

Time/Distance/Totals, if any: _____

6

Date, day, time, location: _____

Feeling of energy/health before: _____*during:*_____ *after:* _____

Challenges: _____

Max effort/breathing/pulse: _____

Core: _____

Stretching: _____

Successes: _____

Other: _____

Time/Distance/Totals, if any: _____

7

Date, day, time, location: _____

Feeling of energy/health before: _____*during:*_____ *after:* _____

Challenges: _____

Max effort/breathing/pulse: _____

Core: _____

Stretching: _____

Successes: _____

Other: _____

Time/Distance/Totals, if any: _____

8

Date, day, time, location: _____

Feeling of energy/health before: _____*during:*_____ *after:* _____

Challenges: _____

Max effort/breathing/pulse: _____

Core: _____

Stretching: _____

Successes: _____

Other: _____

Time/Distance/Totals, if any: _____

9

Date, day, time, location: _____

Feeling of energy/health before: _____*during:*_____ *after:* _____

Challenges: _____

Max effort/breathing/pulse: _____

Core: _____

Stretching: _____

Successes: _____

Other: _____

Time/Distance/Totals, if any: _____

10

Date, day, time, location: _____

Feeling of energy/health before: _____*during:*_____ *after:* _____

Challenges: _____

Max effort/breathing/pulse: _____

Core: _____

Stretching: _____

Successes: _____

Other: _____

Time/Distance/Totals, if any: _____

11

Date, day, time, location: _____

Feeling of energy/health before: _____*during:*_____ *after:* _____

Challenges: _____

Max effort/breathing/pulse: _____

Core: _____

Stretching: _____
Successes: _____
Other: _____
Time/Distance/Totals, if any: _____

12

Date, day, time, location: _____
Feeling of energy/health before: _____*during:*_____ *after:* _____
Challenges: _____
Max effort/breathing/pulse: _____
Core: _____
Stretching: _____
Successes: _____
Other: _____
Time/Distance/Totals, if any: _____

13

Date, day, time, location: _____
Feeling of energy/health before: _____*during:*_____ *after:* _____
Challenges: _____
Max effort/breathing/pulse: _____
Core: _____
Stretching: _____
Successes: _____
Other: _____
Time/Distance/Totals, if any: _____

14

Date, day, time, location: _____
Feeling of energy/health before: _____*during:*_____ *after:* _____
Challenges: _____
Max effort/breathing/pulse: _____
Core: _____
Stretching: _____
Successes: _____
Other: _____
Time/Distance/Totals, if any: _____

What shall I do today . . . heute . . . hoy . . . aujourd'hui . . . oggi . . . idag . . . tanaan . . . avui . . .

15
Date, day, time, location: _____
Feeling of energy/health before: _____during:_____ after: _____
Challenges: _____
Max effort/breathing/pulse: _____
Core: _____
Stretching: _____
Successes: _____
Other: _____
Time/Distance/Totals, if any: _____

16
Date, day, time, location: _____
Feeling of energy/health before: _____during:_____ after: _____
Challenges: _____
Max effort/breathing/pulse: _____
Core: _____
Stretching: _____
Successes: _____
Other: _____
Time/Distance/Totals, if any: _____

17
Date, day, time, location: _____
Feeling of energy/health before: _____during:_____ after: _____
Challenges: _____
Max effort/breathing/pulse: _____
Core: _____
Stretching: _____
Successes: _____
Other: _____
Time/Distance/Totals, if any: _____

18
Date, day, time, location: _____
Feeling of energy/health before: _____during:_____ after: _____
Challenges: _____
Max effort/breathing/pulse: _____
Core: _____

Stretching: _____

Successes: _____

Other: _____

Time/Distance/Totals, if any: _____

19

Date, day, time, location: _____

Feeling of energy/health before: _____during:_____ after: _____

Challenges: _____

Max effort/breathing/pulse: _____

Core: _____

Stretching: _____

Successes: _____

Other: _____

Time/Distance/Totals, if any: _____

20

Date, day, time, location: _____

Feeling of energy/health before: _____during:_____ after: _____

Challenges: _____

Max effort/breathing/pulse: _____

Core: _____

Stretching: _____

Successes: _____

Other: _____

Time/Distance/Totals, if any: _____

21

Date, day, time, location: _____

Feeling of energy/health before: _____during:_____ after: _____

Challenges: _____

Max effort/breathing/pulse: _____

Core: _____

Stretching: _____

Successes: _____

Other: _____

Time/Distance/Totals, if any: _____

22

Date, day, time, location: _____

Feeling of energy/health before: _____*during:*_____ *after:* _____

Challenges: _____

Max effort/breathing/pulse: _____

Core: _____

Stretching: _____

Successes: _____

Other: _____

Time/Distance/Totals, if any: _____

23

Date, day, time, location: _____

Feeling of energy/health before: _____*during:*_____ *after:* _____

Challenges: _____

Max effort/breathing/pulse: _____

Core: _____

Stretching: _____

Successes: _____

Other: _____

Time/Distance/Totals, if any: _____

24

Date, day, time, location: _____

Feeling of energy/health before: _____*during:*_____ *after:* _____

Challenges: _____

Max effort/breathing/pulse: _____

Core: _____

Stretching: _____

Successes: _____

Other: _____

Time/Distance/Totals, if any: _____

25

Date, day, time, location: _____

Feeling of energy/health before: _____*during:*_____ *after:* _____

Challenges: _____

Max effort/breathing/pulse: _____

Core: _____

Stretching: _____

Successes: _____

Other: _____

Time/Distance/Totals, if any: _____

26

Date, day, time, location: _____

Feeling of energy/health before: _____during:_____ after: _____

Challenges: _____

Max effort/breathing/pulse: _____

Core: _____

Stretching: _____

Successes: _____

Other: _____

Time/Distance/Totals, if any: _____

27

Date, day, time, location: _____

Feeling of energy/health before: _____during:_____ after: _____

Challenges: _____

Max effort/breathing/pulse: _____

Core: _____

Stretching: _____

Successes: _____

Other: _____

Time/Distance/Totals, if any: _____

28

Date, day, time, location: _____

Feeling of energy/health before: _____during:_____ after: _____

Challenges: _____

Max effort/breathing/pulse: _____

Core: _____

Stretching: _____

Successes: _____

Other: _____

Time/Distance/Totals, if any: _____

29

Date, day, time, location: _____
Feeling of energy/health before: _____ during: _____ after: _____
Challenges: _____
Max effort/breathing/pulse: _____
Core: _____
Stretching: _____
Successes: _____
Other: _____
Time/Distance/Totals, if any: _____

30

Date, day, time, location: _____
Feeling of energy/health before: _____ during: _____ after: _____
Challenges: _____
Max effort/breathing/pulse: _____
Core: _____
Stretching: _____
Successes: _____
Other: _____
Time/Distance/Totals, if any: _____

31

Date, day, time, location: _____
Feeling of energy/health before: _____ during: _____ after: _____
Challenges: _____
Max effort/breathing/pulse: _____
Core: _____
Stretching: _____
Successes: _____
Other: _____
Time/Distance/Totals, if any: _____

Extra Workouts 1

Date, day, time, location: _____

Feeling of energy/health before: _____during:_____ after: _____

Challenges: _____

Max effort/breathing/pulse: _____

Core: _____

Stretching: _____

Successes: _____

Other: _____

Time/Distance/Totals, if any: _____

Extra 2

Date, day, time, location: _____

Feeling of energy/health before: _____during:_____ after: _____

Challenges: _____

Max effort/breathing/pulse: _____

Core: _____

Stretching: _____

Successes: _____

Other: _____

Time/Distance/Totals, if any: _____

Extra 3

Date, day, time, location: _____

Feeling of energy/health before: _____during:_____ after: _____

Challenges: _____

Max effort/breathing/pulse: _____

Core: _____

Stretching: _____

Successes: _____

Other: _____

Time/Distance/Totals, if any: _____

Extra 4

Date, day, time, location: _____

Feeling of energy/health before: _____during:_____ after: _____

Challenges: _____

Max effort/breathing/pulse: _____

Core: _____

What shall I do today . . . heute . . . hoy . . . aujourd'hui . . . oggi . . . idag . . . tanaan . . . avui . . .

Stretching: _____
Successes: _____
Other: _____
Time/Distance/Totals, if any: _____

Extra 5

Date, day, time, location: _____
Feeling of energy/health before: _____ *during:* _____ *after:* _____
Challenges: _____
Max effort/breathing/pulse: _____
Core: _____
Stretching: _____
Successes: _____
Other: _____
Time/Distance/Totals, if any: _____

End of Month Scoring

Method One: Basic (Number of days I exercised this month):_____

    Ultimate Goal: Every Day

    My Goal for This Month Was: _____

    My Goal for Next Month Is: _____

Method Two: Subtraction (Days I Rowed Minus Days Not):_____

    Initial Goal: Exceed Zero (row at least half the days)

    Ultimate Goal: Same as days in the month.

    My Goal for This Month Was: _____

    My Goal for Next Month Is: _____

Method Three: Division (Percentage = Days Rowed Divided by Total Days): _____

    Ultimate Goal: 100%

    My Goal for This Month Was:_____

    My Goal for Next Month Is: _____

Other Scores and Data for Month (Goals set and met; Times rowed; Distances rowed; Other):

_____

_____

_____

_____

_____

_____

_____

December

"*Inactivity is the main cause of age-related decline in muscle strength and the cross-sectional area of muscles, or muscle mass . . . . Conversely, exercise has been linked to the ability to maintain significant muscle mass and strength.*"
    Encyclopedia, at 588

"*[P]hysical inactivity, especially bed rest during an illness, can greatly worsen the loss [of muscle mass] . . . . [A]fter one day of bed rest, older people may need about 2 weeks of progressively becoming more active to get back to the level of muscle strength they had before bed rest.*"
    Merck, at 13

"*When I was in medical school, in the 1960s, we were taught that you shouldn't exercise people over age forty.*"
    Dr. Kenneth Cooper, Kolata, at 45

"*If your goal is to improve your health, studies in recent years have consistently indicated that you get the most benefit when you go from no exercise at all to exercising moderately.*"
    Kolata, at 262

"*Excessive stress is involved in a wide variety of medical conditions, including heart disease, high blood pressure, ulcers, acid reflux disease, strokes, and many other illnesses. Though most of us have heard that deep breathing can help us relax . . ., many of us do not really know how to breathe deeply.*"
    Dennis Lewis, *Free Your Breath, Free Your Life*, at 159

"*Regular exercise . . . helps keep pulmonary ventilation from decreasing during maximal exercise and hastens recovery following exercise.*"
    Encyclopedia, at 590

"*Despite the aging process, regular exercise training results in a significant improvement in aerobic capacity.*"
    Encyclopedia, at 591-92

December – Diet, Body Weight and Feeling Good at Year End

As you exercise, you will naturally pay more attention to what you eat. You can use the well-known 'Weight-Watchers' method of counting calories and adjusting portions, and that is useful and productive. But you will also come to recognize a difference between comfort food and energy food.

Many of us eat more for comfort than for sustenance, health or energy. Comfort eating means filling up to have that satisfied feeling. It means eating food because it tastes good at the time, even if it does not make you feel better. It may mean consuming empty calories to soak up the caffeine from too much coffee or soft drinks. It includes drinking something alcoholic to calm down at the end of the day. At one level or another, comfort eating is consuming calories for some type of feeling good (call it, perhaps, 'sedentary good') without regard to what it does to weight, energy, or feeling good in an active sense. It is thinking with your taste buds and 'solar plexus cushion' instead of the whole, active body.

In contrast, energy food provides nutrients you need without filling you up. We all know that when we exercise with too much food in the gut we feel weaker, slower and find it harder to breathe deeply. Eat smaller portions, yes, but also skip the dessert and add a salad. Skip the rolls and eat the vegetables. Take vitamins if you wish, but also eat a fresh and varied diet to obtain vitamins and minerals in your food. Try more vegetarian approaches to obtaining adequate protein instead of relying on meat with the fatty tissue it contains. Consider the Mediterranean diet with more olive oil and other foods that have found to be healthful. Check resources like "Eating on the Wild Side" by Jo Robinson for information on the variations in the disease-fighting nutrient content of different foods. The suggestions can go on and on, but the point is simple: Eat to feel energetic rather than full. Enjoy the feeling of being hungry at some point between meals and snacks rather than the fatigue of feeling satiated.

As you develop this awareness, you can make weight loss part of your program and goals if you think you need to lose weight. You will burn more calories through your exercise; reduce caloric intake at the same time and, if what you eat is for energy rather than comfort, you will further enhance your ability to burn yet more calories.

If a particular part of your body seems to have accumulated unwelcome fat, pay attention to your skin-fold thickness there. (And imagine fat growing among the organs and muscles below the skin, not just in that layer you pinch to check skin-fold thickness.) Develop an image you want of body shape and set a goal for the thickness of the fatty layer below the skin that you want. Work toward those goals. You may find that the accumulation of fat is like the loss of muscle mass with age; the older we get the easier it is to accumulate unwanted fat and the harder it is to take it back off.

The point is not to diet to an extreme or to starve off fat. Rather the point is to avoid eating something extra for energy and then having to work harder to burn off those extra calories. Try new, healthy foods. Explore books and online resources for guidelines. Use your progress to help drive you toward your goals. And make the daily exercise part of your program to obtain the shape and weight you want to have while increasing your muscle tone, fitness and energy. And, as you go through the holiday season when you are surrounded by an over-abundance of cookies and other high-calorie dishes and treats, keep in mind that you do not have to deprive yourself entirely. You can use your daily rowing selection to burn more calories and to keep a feeling of energy and well-being.

Ron has worked for years on adjusting his meat and potatoes diet to improve his energy. As he approached 50 years of age and then kept going, he found that a slab of fat would accumulate faster on his gut each year if he eased off his training. He had to work harder and eat smarter in order to avoid carrying too many unwanted additional pounds in the boat, and he did.

Mel is not convinced that changing diet is important for her. She feels she has a healthy diet. She has had vegan friends and sometimes tries their choices when they eat out. She knows that the competitive athletes in her circle pay more attention to what they eat. But for now, her focus is on the exercise itself.

Andie used to go to Weight Watchers but let it slide when she began to exercise more. Now she tries to learn about what foods will give her the best nutritional value and help her recover fully for the next day's row. This year she plans to pay more attention to the timing of her eating in relation to when she works out to see what the effect is for her.

1

Date, day, time, location: _____

Feeling of energy/health before: _____ *during:*_____ *after:* _____

Challenges: _____

Max effort/breathing/pulse: _____

Core: _____

Stretching: _____

Successes: _____

Other: _____

Time/Distance/Totals, if any: _____

2

Date, day, time, location: _____

Feeling of energy/health before: _____ *during:*_____ *after:* _____

Challenges: _____

Max effort/breathing/pulse: _____

Core: _____

Stretching: _____

Successes: _____

Other: _____

Time/Distance/Totals, if any: _____

3

Date, day, time, location: _____

Feeling of energy/health before: _____ *during:*_____ *after:* _____

Challenges: _____

Max effort/breathing/pulse: _____

Core: _____

Stretching: _____

Successes: _____

Other: _____

Time/Distance/Totals, if any: _____

4

Date, day, time, location: _____

Feeling of energy/health before: _____ *during:*_____ *after:* _____

Challenges: _____

Max effort/breathing/pulse: _____

Core: _____

What shall I do today . . . heute . . . hoy . . . aujourd'hui . . . oggi . . . idag . . . tanaan . . . avui . . .

Stretching: _____

Successes: _____

Other: _____

Time/Distance/Totals, if any: _____

5

Date, day, time, location: _____

Feeling of energy/health before: _____ *during:* _____ *after:* _____

Challenges: _____

Max effort/breathing/pulse: _____

Core: _____

Stretching: _____

Successes: _____

Other: _____

Time/Distance/Totals, if any: _____

6

Date, day, time, location: _____

Feeling of energy/health before: _____ *during:* _____ *after:* _____

Challenges: _____

Max effort/breathing/pulse: _____

Core: _____

Stretching: _____

Successes: _____

Other: _____

Time/Distance/Totals, if any: _____

7

Date, day, time, location: _____

Feeling of energy/health before: _____ *during:* _____ *after:* _____

Challenges: _____

Max effort/breathing/pulse: _____

Core: _____

Stretching: _____

Successes: _____

Other: _____

Time/Distance/Totals, if any: _____

8

Date, day, time, location: _____

Feeling of energy/health before: _____*during:*_____ *after:* _____

Challenges: _____

Max effort/breathing/pulse: _____

Core: _____

Stretching: _____

Successes: _____

Other: _____

Time/Distance/Totals, if any: _____

9

Date, day, time, location: _____

Feeling of energy/health before: _____*during:*_____ *after:* _____

Challenges: _____

Max effort/breathing/pulse: _____

Core: _____

Stretching: _____

Successes: _____

Other: _____

Time/Distance/Totals, if any: _____

10

Date, day, time, location: _____

Feeling of energy/health before: _____*during:*_____ *after:* _____

Challenges: _____

Max effort/breathing/pulse: _____

Core: _____

Stretching: _____

Successes: _____

Other: _____

Time/Distance/Totals, if any: _____

11

Date, day, time, location: _____

Feeling of energy/health before: _____*during:*_____ *after:* _____

Challenges: _____

Max effort/breathing/pulse: _____

Core: _____

Stretching: _____

Successes: _____

Other: _____

Time/Distance/Totals, if any: _____

12

Date, day, time, location: _____

Feeling of energy/health before: _____ *during:* _____ *after:* _____

Challenges: _____

Max effort/breathing/pulse: _____

Core: _____

Stretching: _____

Successes: _____

Other: _____

Time/Distance/Totals, if any: _____

13

Date, day, time, location: _____

Feeling of energy/health before: _____ *during:* _____ *after:* _____

Challenges: _____

Max effort/breathing/pulse: _____

Core: _____

Stretching: _____

Successes: _____

Other: _____

Time/Distance/Totals, if any: _____

14

Date, day, time, location: _____

Feeling of energy/health before: _____ *during:* _____ *after:* _____

Challenges: _____

Max effort/breathing/pulse: _____

Core: _____

Stretching: _____

Successes: _____

Other: _____

Time/Distance/Totals, if any: _____

15

Date, day, time, location: _____

Feeling of energy/health before: _____*during:*_____ *after:* _____

Challenges: _____

Max effort/breathing/pulse: _____

Core: _____

Stretching: _____

Successes: _____

Other: _____

Time/Distance/Totals, if any: _____

16

Date, day, time, location: _____

Feeling of energy/health before: _____*during:*_____ *after:* _____

Challenges: _____

Max effort/breathing/pulse: _____

Core: _____

Stretching: _____

Successes: _____

Other: _____

Time/Distance/Totals, if any: _____

17

Date, day, time, location: _____

Feeling of energy/health before: _____*during:*_____ *after:* _____

Challenges: _____

Max effort/breathing/pulse: _____

Core: _____

Stretching: _____

Successes: _____

Other: _____

Time/Distance/Totals, if any: _____

18

Date, day, time, location: _____

Feeling of energy/health before: _____*during:*_____ *after:* _____

Challenges: _____

Max effort/breathing/pulse: _____

Core: _____

What shall I do today . . . heute . . . hoy . . . aujourd'hui . . . oggi . . . idag . . . tanaan . . . avui . . .

Stretching: _____

Successes: _____

Other: _____

Time/Distance/Totals, if any: _____

19

Date, day, time, location: _____

Feeling of energy/health before: _____ during:_____ after: _____

Challenges: _____

Max effort/breathing/pulse: _____

Core: _____

Stretching: _____

Successes: _____

Other: _____

Time/Distance/Totals, if any: _____

20

Date, day, time, location: _____

Feeling of energy/health before: _____ during:_____ after: _____

Challenges: _____

Max effort/breathing/pulse: _____

Core: _____

Stretching: _____

Successes: _____

Other: _____

Time/Distance/Totals, if any: _____

21

Date, day, time, location: _____

Feeling of energy/health before: _____ during:_____ after: _____

Challenges: _____

Max effort/breathing/pulse: _____

Core: _____

Stretching: _____

Successes: _____

Other: _____

Time/Distance/Totals, if any: _____

22

Date, day, time, location: _____

Feeling of energy/health before: _____*during:*_____ *after:* _____

Challenges: _____

Max effort/breathing/pulse: _____

Core: _____

Stretching: _____

Successes: _____

Other: _____

Time/Distance/Totals, if any: _____

23

Date, day, time, location: _____

Feeling of energy/health before: _____*during:*_____ *after:* _____

Challenges: _____

Max effort/breathing/pulse: _____

Core: _____

Stretching: _____

Successes: _____

Other: _____

Time/Distance/Totals, if any: _____

24

Date, day, time, location: _____

Feeling of energy/health before: _____*during:*_____ *after:* _____

Challenges: _____

Max effort/breathing/pulse: _____

Core: _____

Stretching: _____

Successes: _____

Other: _____

Time/Distance/Totals, if any: _____

25

Date, day, time, location: _____

Feeling of energy/health before: _____*during:*_____ *after:* _____

Challenges: _____

Max effort/breathing/pulse: _____

Core: _____

Stretching: _____

Successes: _____

Other: _____

Time/Distance/Totals, if any: _____

26

Date, day, time, location: _____

Feeling of energy/health before: _____ *during:* _____ *after:* _____

Challenges: _____

Max effort/breathing/pulse: _____

Core: _____

Stretching: _____

Successes: _____

Other: _____

Time/Distance/Totals, if any: _____

27

Date, day, time, location: _____

Feeling of energy/health before: _____ *during:* _____ *after:* _____

Challenges: _____

Max effort/breathing/pulse: _____

Core: _____

Stretching: _____

Successes: _____

Other: _____

Time/Distance/Totals, if any: _____

28

Date, day, time, location: _____

Feeling of energy/health before: _____ *during:* _____ *after:* _____

Challenges: _____

Max effort/breathing/pulse: _____

Core: _____

Stretching: _____

Successes: _____

Other: _____

Time/Distance/Totals, if any: _____

29

Date, day, time, location: _____

Feeling of energy/health before: _____during:_____ after: _____

Challenges: _____

Max effort/breathing/pulse: _____

Core: _____ _____

Stretching: _____

Successes: _____

Other: _____

Time/Distance/Totals, if any: _____

30

Date, day, time, location: _____

Feeling of energy/health before: _____during:_____ after: _____

Challenges: _____

Max effort/breathing/pulse: _____

Core: _____

Stretching: _____

Successes: _____

Other: _____

Time/Distance/Totals, if any: _____

31

Date, day, time, location: _____

Feeling of energy/health before: _____during:_____ after: _____

Challenges: _____

Max effort/breathing/pulse: _____

Core: _____

Stretching: _____

Successes: _____

Other: _____

Time/Distance/Totals, if any: _____

Extra Workouts 1

Date, day, time, location: _____

Feeling of energy/health before: _____ *during:* _____ *after:* _____

Challenges: _____

Max effort/breathing/pulse: _____

Core: _____

Stretching: _____

Successes: _____

Other: _____

Time/Distance/Totals, if any: _____

Extra 2

Date, day, time, location: _____

Feeling of energy/health before: _____ *during:* _____ *after:* _____

Challenges: _____

Max effort/breathing/pulse: _____

Core: _____

Stretching: _____

Successes: _____

Other: _____

Time/Distance/Totals, if any: _____

Extra 3

Date, day, time, location: _____

Feeling of energy/health before: _____ *during:* _____ *after:* _____

Challenges: _____

Max effort/breathing/pulse: _____

Core: _____

Stretching: _____

Successes: _____

Other: _____

Time/Distance/Totals, if any: _____

Extra 4

Date, day, time, location: _____

Feeling of energy/health before: _____ *during:* _____ *after:* _____

Challenges: _____

Max effort/breathing/pulse: _____

Core: _____

Stretching: _____

Successes: _____

Other: _____

Time/Distance/Totals, if any: _____

Extra 5

Date, day, time, location: _____

Feeling of energy/health before: _____during:_____ after: _____

Challenges: _____

Max effort/breathing/pulse: _____

Core: _____

Stretching: _____

Successes: _____

Other: _____

Time/Distance/Totals, if any: _____

End of Month Scoring

Method One: Basic (Number of days I exercised this month):_____
    Ultimate Goal: Every Day
    My Goal for This Month Was: _____
    My Goal for Next Month Is: _____
Method Two: Subtraction (Days I Rowed Minus Days Not):_____
    Initial Goal: Exceed Zero (row at least half the days)
    Ultimate Goal: Same as days in the month.
    My Goal for This Month Was: _____
    My Goal for Next Month Is: _____
Method Three: Division (Percentage = Days Rowed Divided by Total Days): _____
    Ultimate Goal: 100%
    My Goal for This Month Was:_____
    My Goal for Next Month Is: _____

Other Scores and Data for Month (Goals set and met; Times rowed; Distances rowed; Other):

_____

_____

_____

_____

_____

_____

Season/Year Recap and Change

Scoring

You have calculated your score at the end of each month. Take a season-long look at your progress and look back at the year, as well. Have you improved during the this season? Compare season to season as the year progresses. Most importantly, once you calculate your score, consider whether it correlates with how you feel.

_____

_____

_____

_____

_____

Goals Accomplished

Look back on your goals for the past season and the year. Did you set goals for your score based on how many days you rowed? Did you set goals to row longer each day? If you are succeeding with both of those challenges, how are you doing at including core work and stretching each day? (Are you recording that?) Do you also set goals for distances rowed or pace? Have you planned to take a rowing class or attend a rowing event? For these and other goals you may have set three months ago, look back and record here how you did.

_____

_____

_____

_____

_____

_____

Goals Looking Ahead

Once you have looked back, plan ahead. Set some goals. Make them realistic based on your past experience, and your other plans for the coming year and the coming season.

_____

_____

_____

_____

_____

Changes for Variety

Do you cross-train for variety? How can you modify that in the coming season? Plan a vacation based on doing something active you would enjoy. Add an aerobics or spinning or Pilates class or some weight lifting or yoga or something else you may not normally do.

_____

_____

_____

_____

_____

Conclusion

Looking Back; Looking Ahead

What worked and what did not:

- Schedule: Have you found ways to fit daily exercise into your work and family schedule? Is it the same every day; every season? What worked for you and what did not?
- Location: Have you settled on where you will row? Are there other opportunities?
- Machine: Are you happy with the equipment you are using? What do you like and not like about it – and can you make changes to address what you do not like?
- Time of day, meals, and interruptions: Is this working well or do you need to step back and consider how to make it work better for you?
- Type of workout (steady state, interval, other; distance and time rowed): Time for an annual review. Look back at the four seasons. Do you want to follow the same progression for the coming year or make some changes? What did you learn?
- Stretching: It is easy to leave out but makes a great difference if you include it. Would a class in stretching help?
- Core work: Same with core work. The front, sides and back of the mid-section require extra attention. Have you made the time and are you satisfied with the results?
- Wind, fitness, muscle tone, ability to succeed at other activities, weight control, health/doctor's exam, other: Make your own list and record your observations for the year. What changes have you seen and what are your goals for the coming year?

_____

_____

_____

_____

What shall I do today . . . heute . . . hoy . . . aujourd'hui . . . oggi . . . idag . . . tanaan . . . avui . . .

Appendices

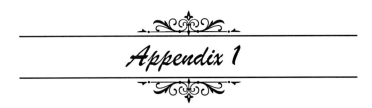

Appendix 1

Why Use a Training Journal or Log

The biggest challenge to achieving a fitness goal is not age or weakness or lack of ability; it is distractions. One reason that setting a goal and keeping a log are the two best ways to exercise daily is that they help provide focus to avoid, or at least work your way past or through, the many distractions.

Do not misunderstand the use of the term "distractions" to imply that what gets in the way of daily exercise is always unimportant. Certainly, some distractions like watching TV or using the computer and mobile devices to 'play' or reading escape literature are not necessarily adding to your life beyond the momentary enjoyment or relaxation you experience while distracted with them. But there are many distractions that are supremely important, such as being with family, making a living and caring for the young, the old, the ill and the infirm. It is relatively rare, however, that even the most important things in life require our attention 24/7 or require that we not row.

Setting a goal helps because it adds purpose to your daily exercise. It may help you get in that seventh row of the week that you otherwise might have foregone. And, along with the memory of your initial fitness, a goal 'bookends' your experience on the rowing machine each day. You not only know where you began; you also can compare it to where you want to end up – at your goal. What you do today is now not just a coin in the fountain but a link in a chain, a step on that path toward the goal, one more day in the weeks or months to the goal. With a goal in mind, you are more likely to see your row today as a means to that end. You will tend to pay attention to what you are doing in a different way. You will be more likely to use your row today to advance your fitness, and that can add to your enjoyment and what you get out of it.

That raises an interesting question: Does it matter what type of goal you set? Your goal may be anything, from rowing for a longer time or greater distance to rowing a particular piece at a specified pace, attending an event, or learning something new. Rowing daily may initially have seemed like an ultimate or unattainable challenge in itself. Once you achieve a routine of daily rowing, however, you will find it provides a strong foundation upon which you can build toward other goals more successfully. (And, conversely, your other goals may make rowing daily feel like a helpful means to a goal rather than an imposing challenge.) Over time you will find that the goals you set evolve with your level of interest, fitness, age and experience.

Each of the other (besides rowing daily) goals you set can help in several ways. A goal to row a longer distance gives you an incentive today to see if you can increase the distance over what you have rowed before. It may also encourage you to learn more about ways to increase that form of stamina (the ability to keep going longer). A goal to row faster will give you an incentive to work on your pace and to experiment with and apply interval training to enhance your speed. You may begin to notice different bodily feedback as to your muscular stamina (when your muscles begin to feel weak) and your wind (when you feel so out of breath that you want to stop). It may cause you to adjust your stroke rate and to pay attention in a different way to the interplay between strength and wind at the different stroke rates you try. A goal of attending an event can add a social, volunteer/contribution or other aspect to your rowing and may lead to your becoming involved in a new way with the rowing community. That, in turn, can pay back to you with dividends as you learn from others.

How does keeping a journal or log to record your daily exercise help improve your fitness? Writing it down does not change what you just did. It does not dictate what you will do tomorrow. But it does involve another form of paying attention that, over time, will tend to enhance your exercise experience. Consider the following three points:

- Knowing you will record what you do can affect what you plan to do;
- Recording observations about the workout may help you pay attention to different aspects of your experience; and
- With a written record, you can look back, see your progress and compare not only how you are doing now but also how different circumstances have affected your exercise and how you felt at the time.

Even if you simply do a 'workout of the day' as defined by someone else, your personal record will give you feedback that is useful to you and, someday, may form the basis for your defining your own workouts.

Achieving a goal and having a record of a year's exercise can both provide satisfaction. Those are worthwhile benefits, too. But my point to you is that the process you engage in as a result of setting goals and keeping a log is, in and of itself, a tremendous benefit in the way it enhances your daily exercise, the exact scope and nature of which will depend on you. There is always more to this than the goal or the log. There is something to be gained even if you do not achieve the goal you set, even if your log is incomplete – or even if you make your goal and begin again. We are not striving for perfection, only to live with more energy and enjoyment. Try it and see what you experience.

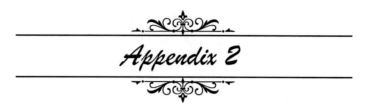

Appendix 2

Coaching: Self-directed or Not?

There is a broad spectrum of options for coaching or otherwise applying training ideas to your daily rowing routine. At one end of the spectrum, simply start rowing without worrying about a regimen, a routine, having a coach or otherwise 'doing it right.' You can always learn more and get coaching later. At the other end of the spectrum, you can find a coach who will study your current condition, consider your goals, and give you a routine with regular feedback to direct how you proceed from point A to point B.

The information in the following appendices is offered for those between those two ends of the spectrum. It is not complete or definitive. It is not intended to help you achieve any particular goal, except to offer some input you can apply according to your preference and your experience.

Keep in mind that other resources exist, other options along the spectrum of training alternatives. These include obtaining guidance or advice from a friend or local rower; taking a rowing class at a health club, gym, or rowing club; and examining plans and workout choices others have offered and picking and choosing what portions of those you think you can productively apply to your own situation.

Use caution. Apply your own judgment based on your experience to the use of any workout you borrow from someone else. There are many reasons borrowing ideas can be helpful:

- You try something new you had not thought of yourself;
- It opens a door to a different range of workouts;
- It helps you past an impasse; or, perhaps,
- It makes you aware of another resource with even more helpful ideas.

There are also many reasons to be cautious when trying to use a workout idea taken from a different context and apply it to yours:

- The information may be incomplete;
- It may have been geared for someone in a very different condition;
- It may be one part of a sequence you are not following;
- It could even be designed to address a particular need of someone else in a different situation.

These are not reasons to avoid learning from others. Share ideas. Experiment. But in the end apply your own judgment as you have developed it based on your experience.

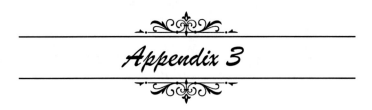

Appendix 3

Training Plans: A General Introduction

Following is a brief summary of information you may find interesting or useful in assessing or adding to your daily rowing if you are not on a training regimen. Please keep in mind the starting admonition (just row; do not wait to 'get it right'). If the information here helps you enjoy and get more out of your rowing, then it has served its purpose. But if it distracts you or causes you to question or limit your rowing, it would be better ignored. In that case, simply go back to rowing each day.

Conversely, if you have a training routine or have followed one before, you may find this to be too basic. It is intended to provide ideas as a starting point. The purpose is to stimulate your thinking if you are proceeding on your own, not to lay out a routine.

A. Rowing Without a Plan

It is day one. You get on the rowing machine without any work out plan. Just as you would do if you were going for a walk, you start out and you move. That in itself is useful and fine to do. A training plan, regimen or goal is not required. Simply moving feels good and is good for the body.

You do not have to exercise to a target or according to a plan in order for it to be beneficial, to gain flexibility, strength and stamina. If the unplanned approach to rowing appeals to you and works for you, stick with it; do not feel you have to set a goal, monitor your speed, control the number of strokes you take per minute, or otherwise manage the experience.

To stay with self-directed or 'unplanned' rowing for a moment longer, you will find if you use this approach that a number of variables may occur from time to time. Just as going for a walk on a given day may take you either around the block or for two miles along the river, your rows may vary in length according to what suits you each day. You may also occasionally feel stronger and row harder or faster. On other days, you may get bored sooner or feel tired more quickly. You may decide on the spur of the moment to pay attention to pace or stroke rate or heart rate or breathing rate or some other aspect of your rowing and/or your body, but that is your choice at the time, not a planned or required or managed activity.

As you row, just as with walking and other informal activities, you will find with a regular routine that you can continue to row for a longer time or distance more easily. Each day you row, the experience will provide cumulative effects, just as if you were adding a child's block to a toy house, a dollar to a bank account or a shovel of snow to a snow bank. Whether you notice it daily or not, the cumulative effect over time will become appreciable. With unplanned rows, you can use that beneficial effect however you choose, whether it be to row longer, row harder, or just enjoy the same row more each day. At some point, you may wish to develop a plan.

B. Adding Elements of a Plan or Structure

Probably the most effective way to approach exercise planning is to find a coach, follow his or her advice, and begin a program that is based on the coach's review of your fitness and developed specifically to help you achieve your goals. Alternatively, you can do a 'row of the day' workout (like Concept2's), study and use rowing workouts (like Lisa Schlenker's "ERG: 75 Workouts for Athletes" [Urban Erg, 2009]) or examine training plans (like Mike Caviston's "Wolverine Plan") and develop your own program which you can then follow day-to-day and month-to-month. You can find resources like Darryl Wilkinson's "Indoor Rowing for Fitness and Competition" (Crowood Press, 2010), in which the author sets forth multi-week "training programmes" for various levels of ability and experience. You can glean ideas from books such as Jim Flood and Charles Simpson's "The Complete Guide to Indoor Rowing," part of a series of 'complete' guides to exercise and training published by Bloomsbury Publishing (2012). And you can use resources like the chapter on "Main Rowing Regimens" in Jay Nithus' "Indoor Rowing: Perfection in Exercise" (2009). You can also find numerous training logs like "Runner's World Training Journal" that contain a variety of advice on exercise and nutrition.

The following ideas are not a guide intended to help you develop a rigorous training program like Lisa Schlenker's or Mike Caviston's. Rather, if you are not working under a coach and not following a carefully laid-out regimen, this information may spur independent thinking and planning on your own, whether that planning is something you do over time, the night before or only as you sit down on the rowing machine to begin.

You may decide to add something to your daily rowing for variety or entertainment, to get faster, to burn more calories, or for other reasons. Your reason may affect what you choose to do. If your goal is to entertain yourself, to make the daily row more painless or to fit it into your otherwise full routine more seamlessly, you may choose to watch TV while you row or take on another element that serves that end. If your goal is to burn more calories, you will likely select options that lengthen your row, speed up your pace or both.

If you exercise based on how you feel today, you will not plan in advance what you will do but only that you will row. Set aside sufficient time to row 30-60 minutes and to include some stretching and core work after you row. When you are ready to begin rowing, either simply sit down and begin to row or take a moment to decide what you feel like doing that day. You can take into consideration whether you feel strong or weak, energetic or tired, focused or distracted. Over time, you will be able to decide what workouts will make the best use of how you are feeling so that you complete the exercise and advance to the next day in the best position to continue to make progress over time.

It is common as someone exercises more than they used to for them to reach a point where the limiting factor seems to be either the wind or the muscles. If the muscles seem sore or weak and that is holding you back, focus on developing them. For example, if your arms or back tire first as you row, that may be because they are weaker than your legs and/or that your technique is putting an undue burden on them in relation to your legs. Work on your technique to relax the arms and to use the body/back efficiently. It may help to do some exercises to strengthen the arms or the core. Later, work on the legs. On the other hand, if your limiting factor seems to be your wind, use interval work or other activities to challenge your wind: Get winded today to gain wind tomorrow.

If you decide the unplanned approach is boring or ineffective, you may want structure to design a routine or to give yourself something to focus on while rowing. A plan or structure may also provide a tool for comparing one row to another. And a plan can provide your goal for the day; rowing to the plan can provide the satisfaction of meeting that goal.

There are many ways to incorporate a small amount of planning into your daily rows without creating a detailed workout regimen:

- Take a Break: After rowing a little, take a break. Get a drink of water and start again instead of putting the machine away;
- Time: Whatever time you rowed yesterday, add five minutes;
- Stroke Rate and Power: As you row, try to reduce your stroke rate while keeping the pace the same;
- Distance: Whatever distance you rowed yesterday, round up to the next significant figures or just add 500 meters;
- Unit of Measure: If you usually row with the meters setting, try it on calories or watts;
- Media: Using the radio or TV, row throughout a particular show or segment;

- Music: Same idea – row through certain songs, an album, a movement of a symphony or part of an opera;
- Winded: Row until you feel winded. Then, instead of stopping, slow down but keep going;
- Not Winded: After you have rowed until you feel warmed up but not winded, take up the pace until you feel winded. Try this with a higher stroke rate; then try it with leg power at a low stroke rate instead of raising the rate.
- Ask another rower what she likes to do for an enjoyable row and try it;
- Review your record of past rows and pick one to repeat and improve on, with a goal for the re-row;
- From books and online resources about rowing, select a workout and try it;
- And the range of your options goes on and on.

Injecting an element of intentional planning like these may suit you and provide all the structure or regimen you need or want. If you feel you want more, read on and consider developing a multi-day plan.

C. Creating Your Own Basic Plan

You decide that you want to have a plan or organizational structure to follow. The ultimate exercise plan may be one with a scheduled workout that tells you precisely what to do each day for the week (or month or longer). I am not offering that here. You could develop that or you could make arrangements with a coach to provide you a detailed exercise plan. It might be tailored to your fitness and needs and goals. Or it might simply be a model for you to follow.

The following, instead, is some information you can use to decide for yourself what you will do day to day or week by week. The decision is yours. The process you follow can be as planned or as spur of the moment as you wish.

1. Select a time period to use as your basic unit for a series of workouts you will repeat. It could be one or two weeks, for example.
2. Consider resources you may want to rely on or be able to use, such as written or online input, a friend's advice, or generalized suggestions from a coach at the local boathouse.
3. Consider possible choices for workouts (see the following appendices regarding steady state and interval options).
4. Use flexibility as you implement your plan. Remember, the first goal is to row each day; until you develop that habit, the rest of this should serve that end, not get in the way of it.
5. At the end of each unit of time, review and revise what you have planned. Repeat with modifications.
6. If you find a routine that suits you and your schedule, follow it for as long as suits you.

7. If you need to make a change, simply do a different row. This situation may arise with illness, travel and other types of conflict. Once you clear the conflict, you can choose whether to go back to the routine or modify it.
8. Do what works for you.

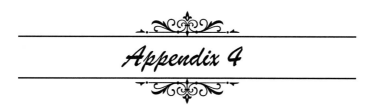

Appendix 4

Steady State Workouts

A 'steady state' row is simply one you do at a steady pace, a pace that is approximately even without deliberate and substantial changes. The pace does not have to remain exactly the same or meet particular criteria. For example, the pace may be faster or slower. The time may be short or long. The stroke rate may be low or high. The point is that, taking into consideration that you may spend some time warming up and your pace may vary according to how you feel (from ups and downs based on feeling strong mid-piece to gradually increasing your pace as you approach the finish), the pace will generally be 'steady' or approximately 'even' from start to finish. The point is not that you must maintain precise uniformity. Rather, "steady" simply contrasts with interval work (see the next appendix), in which you deliberately row harder for selected intervals and alternate those with easier or lighter intervals.

To illustrate, consider these rowers:

- Tony rows 5k every other day and cycles other days. When he rows, Tony pays attention to pace per 500 meters and his total time. His pace varies in different ways on different days. He pays attention to when he feels warmed up and notices his pace improves during that time, but he does not set target paces or times for himself and he does not do sprints or 'power 10's.'
- Joe usually lifts weights or uses the stair master or elliptical trainer, but some days he rows for 5 minutes as a warm-up before the rest of his workout. He rows at a pace he feels is rowing hard, breaks a sweat pretty quickly, but does not keep track of pace or distance rowed.
- Jackie began rowing 5-10 minutes a day a few weeks ago. Initially, she felt little resistance and no noticeable change day to day. Eventually, she began to extend the time she rowed. She began to set a target time (20 minutes, later 30 minutes) and tried to row farther in each given time than she had the day before. Some days she would set the monitor to record her progress in calories rather than meters. She began to notice change.

- Ellen had rowed on the river in a learn-to-row class the previous spring. They were on the water for an hour. She figured she could row 10k in an hour or less and set the monitor for that distance. Now she is working on reducing the amount of time it takes to row that distance.
- Steve puts on the news, turns up the volume and rows. He just lets the monitor kick into gear without any settings and does not pay attention to it. At the end of the news, he records the number of meters he has rowed, figuring he may want to review it someday, but with no distance or speed goals.
- Sandy is training for a race several months away. She begins pieces of varying length (from 5k to 15k) and time (from 20 minutes to 80 minutes) by pushing hard right away to warm up, hitting a pace slightly faster than she expects to maintain for the full time or distance. She then watches the monitor for the rest of the row. Her two goals each time she rows are to start a little faster and to keep the pace from rising as much as it did the last time she did that piece.

All of these rowers are essentially rowing steady state. Some would argue that a very short row does not count or otherwise suggest ways several of these rowers could get more out of the experience. And some coaches would describe steady state rowing as longer pieces at a lower stroke rate. But there is something all these examples have in common: Accepting that there may be some variation for warming up, warming down or natural changes of pace during the body of the row, all of these rowers are rowing at a relatively even or steady pace during the body of their pieces, as opposed to deliberately changing the pace or level of effort in a dramatic way.

The level of effort you apply during a steady state row can be anything from minimal to high. For example, Sandy may be using her pieces to push her anaerobic threshold. You would have to talk with her to find out. When she sets her starting pace and then tries to hold it, how out of breath is she and how soon does it begin? Is her body telling her she should slow down or stop at any point, throughout the piece, or not at all? She could be rowing at her limit, pushing her anaerobic threshold, or she could be setting a comfortable pace she could maintain all day if she did not have other things to do. But her goal and her practice is to maintain a roughly even pace.

Steady state rowing is, to many people, what seems natural. Rowing 'pieces,' doing 'power 10s,' taking the stroke up, and other actions that disrupt a steady pace all may feel unwelcome to some rowers. And you can row steady state at varying speeds and for different distances and using different stroke rates, thus allowing a substantial training component. You can break a sweat, get out of breath, burn calories, improve your health, and improve your fitness. Or you can simply row just as you would simply walk or jog. It all helps.

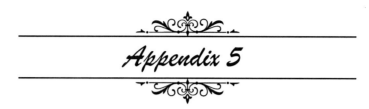

Appendix 5

Interval Workouts

Rowing intervals contrasts with steady state rowing because doing intervals involves rowing harder than your usual or relaxed pace for a relatively short period of time or distance and then rowing more easily to recover, before repeating the more intense interval, and so on. It is a deliberate, planned workout that involves rowing a selected number of intervals harder for selected times or distances, with pre-determined rest (slower pace – not stopping) in between the harder intervals.

For a competitive athlete in training, the harder intervals would usually be rowed at full pressure and the rest intervals at a paddle or light pressure. The difference would be tremendous.

For many of us who are not in as great condition, whether due to lack of training or other reasons, the difference between power and rest will not be as great, but it will be significant to us. Since part of the benefit of doing intervals comes from that difference, if you find that you can create a greater distinction between power and rest with shorter pieces, go for it. Consider it a way to simulate the muscle-building benefits of lifting weights, a way to incorporate resistance training into your routine.

A short interval may be only a few strokes. One of the easiest and most basic interval workouts, for example, is to row 10 strokes "on" (at power) and 10 or more "off" (recovering), repeating those two (10 on-10 off) for as long as you want. In fact, a great series of workouts you can undertake over a period of days or weeks, if you are out of condition and looking to improve, is to row a set distance doing 10s at power without counting the number of strokes it takes to recover between power 10s (presumably more than 10 easy strokes, at least at first). Instead, count the number of power 10s you can row in that set distance or time. For example, you might row fifteen 10s in five kilometers with varying amounts of rest between each that you measure only by when you 'catch your breath' and are ready for the next "power ten." Then, over a series of days rowing the same distance, see how many more power 10s you can row in that distance. Increasing the number will correspondingly decrease the rest between 10s because the total distance is the same. (You may be pleasantly surprised to learn how easy it is over a period of days to improve this measure of your fitness.)

There can be as many possible intervals as there are minutes on the clock and distances you can measure. The usual practice is that, if you are rowing shorter intervals, you row more of them; if you are rowing longer intervals, you row fewer. So, for example, you might row three 2,000 meter pieces with rest in between, but six or eight 1,000 meter pieces, eight to twelve 500 meter pieces, and so on. Or, if you are measuring power intervals by time, you might row three ten minute pieces, six or more five minute pieces, 10 or more two minute pieces, and so on.

Another aspect of rowing intervals is selecting a useful rest period between the power intervals. Coaches will treat the rest interval timing as just as important as the length of the power intervals. You may choose to establish rest intervals that serve your goal of recovering your wind between pieces or some other target such as a particular pulse. If you are rowing very long intervals, you will likely find that you do not want your rest to match the power piece in length. On the other hand, if your intervals are shorter, you may extend the rest time or distance to match the power interval in duration or select another rest period that works for you.

As you can see, you can play with rowing intervals to create a wide variety of different workouts. The general goal they will all have in common is to provide a convenient mechanism by which you can row harder or with more power for a relatively short interval than you would row if you were proceeding to do the whole row steady state. The shorter duration in which you exert greater power is, somewhat like lifting weights, a technique to challenge your muscles and wind, thereby stimulating each to improve day-to-day so that, as time goes by, you become stronger and have better endurance. While similar improvement can be achieved with gradually ratcheting up the pressure over time with steady state rows, you may find that the variety and brevity of intervals gives you an incentive and an opportunity to use the body's natural adaptive capability more easily than with a long intense row. (More on the subject of will power at another time.)

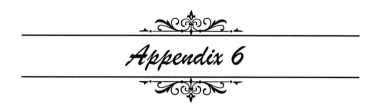

Appendix 6

Combining Intervals with Steady State

The two preceding appendices were basic introductions. They did not get into detail. They did not lay out a universe of choices. You can try what makes sense to you and see what works for you. Similarly, the following is more an illustration than a recipe. It is not intended to be complete or to outline a preferred approach, but simply to illustrate what you can do in mixing alternative approaches to rowing each day.

As you can imagine, combining two types of workouts, each of which has multiple options, offers a large number of possible combinations. Some people base their plan on a weekly routine; some use a two- or three-week routine. Whichever you select, within your time frame you can mix and match different types and lengths of pieces (steady state and interval) using a variety of plans.

Here is a sample of what a one-week routine could look like; begin with fewer, longer pieces and work toward shorter intervals, followed by rest and steady state:

- Monday: 3 x 2k or 3 x 10 minutes;
- Tuesday: 6 x 1k or 6 x 5 minutes;
- Wednesday: 8 x 500m or 8 x 2 minutes;
- Thursday: 10 strokes on/10 off or pyramids;
- Friday: Long, easy recovery row;
- Saturday: Test piece(s), for example, if you are targeting an event or want to establish a baseline;
- Sunday: Long steady state piece.

If you are just beginning to establish a regimen for yourself, try fewer or shorter intervals each day. Give yourself a few weeks to see how you like the routine and what it does for you. Feel free to vary it week to week, if you prefer.

An alternative series with more focus on steady state rowing might be:

- Monday: 45 minutes steady state, rowing firmly;
- Tuesday: 2 x 20-30 minutes steady state;
- Wednesday: 3 x 2k;
- Thursday: 6 x five minutes;
- Friday: 12-20 x two minutes;
- Saturday: 5k warm-up, followed by 6k of 10s;
- Sunday: Long steady state recovery piece.

A completely different approach would be to take one type of interval and use it exclusively, alternating with steady state rows, to see how your body responds to it. For example:

- Monday: 30 minutes doing 10 strokes on and easy off (until you catch your breath);
- Tuesday: 45 minutes recovery (easy) row;
- Wednesday: 2k warm-up followed by same as Monday;
- Thursday: 30 minute recovery row;
- Friday: 5k warm-up followed by same as Monday;
- Saturday: 20 minutes of 10 on and as close to 10 strokes off as you can do, followed by 2k warm-down;
- Sunday: Long steady state piece.

Try it for a couple of weeks and see how many more power 10s you can do during the 30 minutes of intervals. If you are satisfied, try the same for longer periods, increase the 10-stroke power pieces to 20-stroke pieces, or use longer intervals. See how you feel with that.

You can see that your selection of number of pieces and the length of each can offer you a large number of combinations. You may want to develop a routine that you follow every week or every two weeks. Or you may wish to vary it from week to week. Combining different intervals, mixing those with steady state rows, adjusting rest times, factoring in stroke rate, and more, all these are aspects of your rowing regimen you can consider and adjust. And for each of them, you can obtain input from coaches, other rowers and on-line resources, as well as from observing your own experience. You will learn over time what works for you.

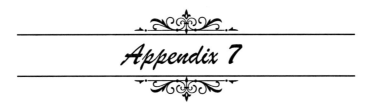

Appendix 7

Level of Effort

"Row within your comfort zone."

What does that mean? To some, the term 'comfort zone' sounds like it should involve only minimal activity, perhaps with snacks or hors d'ouevres and a glass of wine. Consider in the context of moderate exercise that the term is used for a range of exertion you would want to repeat the next day, not a row that was so hard you want to avoid doing it again.

The 'comfort zone' can mean many things:

- I am rowing as hard or as easily as I want to at the time;
- I am comfortable based on my breath, my pulse, my feeling of fatigue, how readily I recover, whether I am enjoying myself, my ability to continue indefinitely (whatever measure feels helpful);
- I do not feel a need to stop;
- I can speak comfortably (or sing along with the music?) while rowing;
- It feels like taking a walk or riding a bike to relax;
- And so on.

The comfort zone can accommodate a wide range of effort. The comfort zone will not include rowing all out and trying to keep going at that pace (except for the very few and very fit whose goal is to do just that on the day in question). But your comfort zone may include rowing harder than normal for a relatively short period, such as doing short intervals with adequate rest between the hard intervals. It may include rowing much harder today than you rowed or could have rowed six months or a year before. It could involve developing so much better wind that it is pleasurable to row out of breath because you know you can keep it up without pain or discomfort.

You can use several different measures to guide the boundaries of your comfort zone:

- The erg monitor: use it for pace and for the time and distance rowed;
- Heart rate monitor: keep track of your pulse as you row and compared to other rows;
- Your breathing: are you taking one or two breaths per stroke; are you breathing more deeply; and do you feel comfortably winded or uncomfortably winded?

One of the challenges of rowing only steady state is that some people find it difficult to row harder and, thus, to increase their strength. Instead, they feel stuck rowing at the same relatively easy or slow pace. That is fine if it is your goal. But if you want to get in better condition or burn more calories, you will want to increase your pace or level of effort one way or another. In some ways, it may actually be easier to row harder intervals interspersed with easier recovery intervals than to push harder over the whole, longer row. And, over time, the effect of the greater resistance you create rowing intervals is to increase your strength. Increased strength allows you to row faster more easily during your steady state rows. In this way, you can expand your comfort zone. At the same time, if you prefer rowing at a steady pace, you can work with that over time and, as your strength and fitness increase, you can row harder but still do so steadily.

Most importantly, use your log to keep track of what you have done. Compare your level of effort over time. You may describe it with pace or time or distance, or with pulse, breathing or other measures. See what is meaningful and works for you.

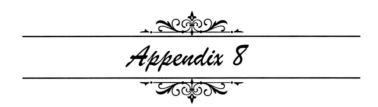

Appendix 8

Rowing Coaches Discuss Training

Kathy and Jules sat in their favorite booth at Rose's Café. Jules was on his first cup of coffee. Formerly a boat builder, Jules had stayed in touch with rowing in the years since he sold the business and went to law school, in part, by meeting with friends at Rose's on the way into the law office.

Two of his oldest friends, Hal and Vinnie, were head coaches of rowing programs at competing colleges in town. Although their styles and personalities were very different, their programs had both enjoyed substantial success over the years. They were regulars at Rose's along with Jules.

More recently, Sarah and Kathy had joined Jules, Vinnie and Hal. They were now regulars, as well. Sarah was older than Kathy. Following a successful college rowing and coaching career, Sarah had switched to using indoor rowing to train rowers and non-rowers alike. She had opened an indoor rowing-centered health club and spent most of her time there. In the summer, she took some of her charges out on the water for training in singles.

Kathy was younger than Sarah. She had been coaching the varsity women at the state university in town for just a couple of years, having moved up from the assistant coach position where she had coached the freshman women. She had rowed for Sarah as an undergrad and now enjoyed meeting with her mentor and the others when she could.

Kathy was warming her hands on her coffee mug, still recovering from the fall chill on the river during her long morning practice. In order to get her rowers back to the boathouse in time to make it to their early classes, Kathy had been on the river with the team almost as early that morning as the baker had been in the kitchen here at Rose's making their signature muffins. Although one muffin could be a meal in itself for some people, Kathy was nibbling on her second muffin of the day, blueberry. With the others not yet to Rose's, Kathy and Jules were still the sole occupants of the large booth where they met and talked most mornings.

"You were saying you were frustrated with your coxswains this morning?" asked Jules.

"Not just the coxswains," said Kathy. "With the whole squad. I had told the coxswains before practice that quick turnaround was critical for the rest periods I wanted them to have between the intervals I wanted them to row. But it was like I had never mentioned it. They sat. They chatted. Rowers took off sweats, chatted and changed foot stretchers between pieces." She looked up and waved as Sarah entered the café.

Jules nodded to Sarah and turned back to Kathy. "So, long delays were a problem, huh?"

Sarah hung her jacket on the hook and sat down next to Kathy. Like Kathy, Sarah had also just finished coaching. But since she trained individuals on indoor rowing machines at her health club, she had not been out in the chill morning like Kathy. And her facility was only a couple of doors down the street from Rose's.

Kathy smiled at Sarah and went on with Jules. "You know, the coxswains did great yesterday when we did long steady state rows out to the end of the basin and back. The coxies in all the eights were focused, kept the stroke rate down, stayed with one another. The rowers kept pulling the whole way, stayed together. And the swing! The girls were commenting afterwards about how great the boats felt, especially during the second half of the long row back. Now that was concentration and team work the way I like it!"

Sarah added cream to her coffee and squeezed Kathy's arm. "You are so lucky to have that experience. We never get to talk about 'swing' on the rowing machines!"

"But today!" said Kathy, and she just shook her head. "I know the problem is the rowers, but I expect the coxies to keep better control."

"Did you get in all the intervals you wanted?" asked Jules.

"Yes, but only because I planned for a very short workout!" Kathy refilled her cup as Hal and Vinnie walked in and came over to the booth.

To some college rowers in town, it would have been odd to see these two together, visiting like old friends. They coached rival men's varsity crews. Their rowers took the rivalry seriously. The coaches understood the rivalry. But, despite that, Hal and Vin had long enjoyed being able to share coaching experiences over coffee at Rose's. They went way back with Jules; and Kathy and Sarah had been welcome additions to the group.

"Hey, Kath," said Hal, having overheard her last comment as they approached. "I saw you launch out on the river long before my guys had their oars on the dock and you were still doing pieces when we brought the boats in. That's a short workout?"

Kathy explained her frustration, pausing only for Betty, their favorite waitress, to take orders for bagels and eggs. When she was done, Vinnie chimed in.

"I've had the same problem, so don't feel bad!" Vinnie said. "I can remember one time the delays were so bad that I sent the other boat ahead on its own to do another pair of pieces out and back while we waited for someone in the other boat. Eventually, I decided I had to choose between two goals. Did I need to have them do the number of pieces I planned, or was the timing of the rest intervals in the workout the key thing I cared the most about?"

Hal smiled. "Knowing you, Vin, I suspect your primary focus was the timing of the intervals. Am I right?"

"Absolutely. Well, the primary focus after how hard they pulled." Vinnie smiled as he held up his cup and nodded gratefully toward Betty as she walked over with another pot of coffee. Then he turned back to Kathy.

"I know you are trying to follow a plan. And that's a good thing," he said, holding up a hand as Kathy began to respond. "But I have watched your rowers since you have been there and I think there is an even more critical thing you are doing than guiding the number and length of pieces of they do."

Hal agreed even before Vinnie could explain what that thing was. "You spend time with them every day focusing on improving their technique, individually and as a boat. I have seen you talking with them."

"Exactly," agreed Vin. "Probably the two most critical contributions you make as a coach are to be able to see what is not right and to get them to correct it. Many coaches simply don't have those skills like you do."

"And they are college kids; they are not going to be focused all the time, especially during an early morning practice after a night of studying late," said Sarah. "There will be better days."

"And, in the meantime, they are the fastest women's crew in the area," said Jules.

"Right," said Kathy gratefully. "But they can be faster still with better attention to their interval work."

The discussion went back to using different distances for intervals and which landmarks along the river were helpful for marking end points or serving as guides for the coxswains. Before they knew it, Betty had delivered their meals. The discussion continued and Kathy seemed to relax as she realized every one of them had days like hers had been. Half an hour later, they were on their way out the door to their offices.

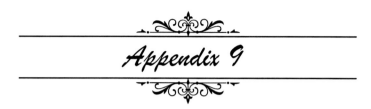

Appendix 9

References and Selected Resources

<u>Selected References, including sources of some quotations:</u>

Beers, Mark H., MD, Editor-in-Chief. *The Merck Manual of Health and Aging.* Merck Research Laboratories, Whitehouse Station, NJ. (2004).

Blech, Joerg. *Healing Through Exercise: Scientifically Proven Ways to Prevent and Overcome Illness and Lengthen Your Life.* Da Capo Press, Cambridge, MA. (English Translation 2009).

Kolata, Gina. *Ultimate Fitness: The Quest for Truth about Exercise and Health.* Farrar, Straus and Giroux, New York, N.Y. (2003).

Kozak, Chrys. Yoga for Rowers. www.yogaforrowers.com. (2009).

Lewis, Dennis. *Free Your Breath, Free Your Life.* Shambhala Publications, Boston, MA. (2004).

Robinson, Jo, *Eating on the Wild Side: The Missing Link to Optimum Health.* Little, Brown & Company, New York, N.Y. (2013).

Rosen, Richard. *The Yoga of Breath: A Step-by-Step Guide to Pranayama,* Shambhala Publications, Boston (2002).

Rowe, John W., M.D., and Kahn, Robert L., Ph.D., *Successful Aging,* Random House, New York (1998).

What shall I do today . . . heute . . . hoy . . . aujourd'hui . . . oggi . . . idag . . . tanaan . . . avui . . .

Zumerchik, John, Editor. *Encyclopedia of Sports Science*, Volume 2, (1997).

For occasional selected references on rowing, rowing equipment, workouts, logs, rowing camps, and more, go to *www.rowdaily.com*. Also, at www.rowdaily.com, you can offer comments and questions and contact the author.

CPSIA information can be obtained
at www.ICGtesting.com
Printed in the USA
FFOW02n1337220415
12859FF